DR. SEBI VS
DR. ENQI

ElectroChemistry ElectroChemistry
Acid-Base Reactions

Chase Duquesnay
EnQi ReaL

Amazon

ISBN: 9798326217745

Cover design by: Enqi ReaL

Printed in the United States of America

FUTURE HOLISTIC SCIENTISTS

CONTENTS

INTRODUCTION

Spelt is a Hybrid.... Lmao!!!

If you can say that out loud, without lightning striking you, then it may be safe for you to read this book. If you get a knee jerk reaction, anxiety, or worse, angry... This book may be the "mental medisin" you need!

There is no way that I could discuss Acids and Alkalines, without dealing with the elephant in the room.

Yes Dr. Sebi recommended Hybrids, Ate Meat, chased very young ladies, robbed banks etc... He was also a Holistic Prophet for many of us, many of us are still standing on his shoulders today.

The thing is there is a difference between standing on his shoulders vs hanging off his back! We have to advance the research!

I may be biased but I don't think anyone has advanced this science like the Melanin vs Daibetes Family... send your support to $MINISTERENQI

H1 O2 N3 C4
BONDS

Your Mind is your Soul, Attention is how you build it. - Dr. EnQi ReaL N.D., M.H., C.P.T., C.S.N., E.C.S., C.P.N.C.

If we join two pieces, one of lead, and the other of silver, so that the two edges join, and if we approach them with the tongue we will feel some taste, quite similar to the taste of vitriol of iron [iron(II) sulfate], while each piece apart gives no trace of this taste. It is not probable that through this junction of the two metals, any solution of one or the other occurs, and that the dissolved particles penetrate the tongue. We must therefore conclude that the junction of these metals produces in one or the other, or in both, a vibration in their particles, and that this vibration, which must necessarily affect the nerves of the tongue, produces there the taste mentioned.
—Johann Georg Sulzer, "Recherches sur l'origine des sentimens agréables et désagréables: Troisième partie. Des plaisirs des sens" 1752

We live in a State of Oxidation, a Oxidation State.

State - the particular condition that someone or something is in at a specific time, a physical condition as regards internal or molecular form or structure, a nation or territory considered as an organized political community under one government, present or introduce (a theme or melody) in a music composition.

Oxidation - Combinaison (d'un corps) avec l'oxygène, donnant un oxyde ; réaction dans laquelle un atome ou un ion perd des électrons, defined as a process that occurs when atoms or groups of atoms lose electrons or when a chemical species gains oxygen or **loses hydrogen**.

Oxidation is gaining Oxygen and losing Hydrogen. Hmmmmm.... Drying out is oxidation. Stay wet, the end. Lmao!

That does make you look at eating fat differently. Insulators are typically thought of as keeping in the electricity but we are starting to get a different picture here. Water is a Nucleophile, the Nucleophile. Water is the Electricity. Ion rich Water. Interesting. Alkaline is Water, the scam is buying Alkaline Water... Natural Water, the Perfect Water should be around 7.6 - 8.6 tops.... Your blood needs to be 7.365 so the water needs to slightly higher to level off. This is has to be based (pun intended) on mineral elements & bicarbonates.

We have to do what has never been done before, Acid-Base & Redox Chemistry. It is insane that this is true but, this is true.

Geometry is it's own Proof.

God is Music.

Body Heat Is ReaL Light....

All that but uh.... Time to do the Math on Project Bowman.

Acid-Alkaline Chemistry is the basis for understanding

all chemical reactions, I would say life itself. Dr. Sebi was the GOAT until...

We will always love him for what he did comma however... Dr. Sebi said Protein is a myth, shame on him. The main purpose of consuming alkaline food is to feed your protein, to maintain your Deoxyribonucleic **Acid** (DNA) health, keep your enzymes active! Please go back and read or reread Melanin vs Diabetes Book 4 the Carbon Edition.

BASEHEADS

Smoking that base...

You didn't know that Crack was Alkaline did you?

Water is a Nucleophile

Cocaine is a Weak Base

Baking Soda is a Weak Base, Baking soda or sodium bicarbonate $NaHCO_3$ is a salt of strong base sodium hydroxide and weak carbonic acid and thus it is a basic salt with a slightly bitter taste. When dissolved in water, there is a formation of sodium hydroxide and carbonic acid that further break down into water and carbon dioxide.

Clearly everything that is "Alkaline" is not healthy for you then, check?

Weak Acid - A weak acid is an acid that partially dissociates into its ions in an aqueous solution or water. Acetic acid, CH3COOH, is a typical weak acid, and it is the ingredient of vinegar. It is partially ionized in its solution. *Proof that you should not consume Apple Cider Vinegar!

Strong Acid - A strong acid is one that is completely dissociated or ionized in an aqueous solution, the factor that decides the classification of strong acids is their ability to release hydrogen ions (H+) into a given solution, strong acids:

1. Chloric acid: $HClO_3$
2. Hydrobromic acid: HBr
3. Hydrochloric acid: HCl
4. Hydroiodic acid: HI
5. Nitric acid: HNO_3
6. Perchloric acid: $HClO_4$
7. Sulfuric acid: H_2SO_4

Weak Base - Ammonia, Copper hydroxide, Aluminium hydroxide, Methylamine, Zinc hydroxide and Lead hydroxide are the 6 weak bases, substances that do not completely dissociate into their constituent ions when dissolved in solutions, their solutions are bad conductors of electricity, they are considered weak electrolytes.

Base - substances that dissolve in water to produce OH- ions and are molecules or ions which are able to accept a hydrogen ion from an acid. A base is any substance that **has a bitter taste**, feels slippery to the touch, and causes colour changes of red litmus paper to blue.

That's why you need to order your bitters now from AmericanHealer.Website

Strong Base - Strong bases are defined as chemical substances that behave like bases and dissociate completely into their respective ions. Many strong bases are metal hydroxides, they are composed of a metal ionically bonding with a **hydroxyl ion** (OH).

Conjugate - a compound formed by the joining of

two or more chemical compounds, become temporarily united in order to exchange genetic material (sex), coupled, connected, or related, a substance formed by the reversible combination of two or more others, a mathematical value or entity having a reciprocal relation with another.

All acids have a conjugate base. All bases have a conjugate acid.

Conjugate Base - A conjugate base is basically an acid that lost its hydrogen ion, a conjugate base is a substance formed by the removal of a proton from an acid.

Conjugate Acid - a conjugate acid is a base that has accepted a proton, a conjugate acid is a substance formed by the removal of an electron from a base or addition of a proton.

The key to Acid-Base Reactions is - Charge Stability.

- Charge Stability is a simply how stable a charge is attached to a particular Atom or Ion.

Was Dr. Sebi a liar or just salesman?

According to Victor Bowman, he was a snake powder salesman lol…

Clearly there was some sexual deviance there because Victor sent me D!@k Pics… Unsolicited of course lol…

"When you breakdown our body, our biological structure, into what we would have to put in it, chemistry, biochemistry. Melanin has no place, its not to be found in the body, that which is attributed to melanin is carbon" - Dr. Sebi

Victor didn't like that I was educating people where

his father fell short, as I continue to do. This is truly what Dr. Sebi would have wanted. Let's get back to that, educating the people.

The key to Acid-Base Reactions is - Charge Stability.
- Charge Stability is a simply how stable a charge is attached to a particular Atom or Ion.

How   do   you   figure   that   out?

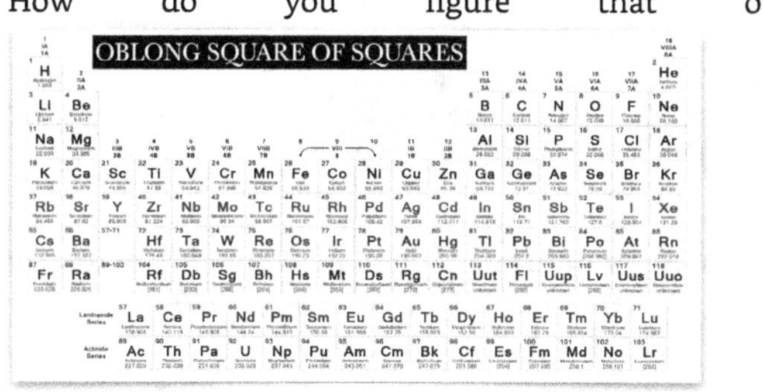

The periodic table functions as a compass of sorts for chemical reactions. - Charge Stability is based on comparison, one atom vs another. Electron stability increases as you go to the Right. The column all the way to the right has the **<u>STRONGEST ATTRACTION</u>** for electrons. This is called electronegativity.

Electronegativity - a chemical property that describes the tendency of an atom or a functional group to attract electrons toward itself, serves as a simple way to quantitatively estimate the **bond energy**, a **measure** of an atom's ability to attract electrons (or electron density) toward itself.

This is where we needed to build to, so we could have

deeper discussions. Have you ever heard of Melanoidins? In the first chapter I mention that bio-electricity is water right? I mentioned drying out being equal to acidifying, death. Fluorine is the most electronegative Adam of them all, the last column is noble gases, they don't react much. They are "bougie"... The Upper Class, they don't mingle.

Fluorine though will steal your girl, like Drake. Drake is having beef with all the rappers and singers because he steals their girls. Drake is Fluorine. Fluorine steals electrons. Only Iodine can really bully fluorine around, this is the thing **<u>NONE OF THE "HOLISTIC HEALERS" know</u>**!

The columns going to the right establish strength, but moving down the column also is a thing... This is why we specifically formulate our Bleu Magick on AmericanHealer.Website like no one else!!! We are fighting Melanoidins!

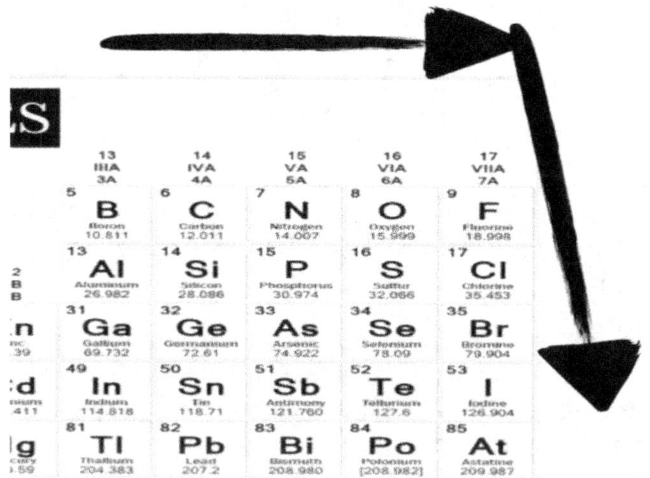

When you move down the table you get larger and larger Atoms, **size does matter**! LMAO…

Did you know that Vitamin A works with Iodine?

In humans there are 3 different iodopsins (rhodopsin analogs) that contain the protein-pigment complexes photopsin I, II, and III.

The 3 types of iodopsins:

Erythrolabe (photopsin I + retinal)

Chlorolabe (photopsin II + retinal)
Cyanolabe (photopsin III + retinal)

These photopsins have absorption maxima for red ["erythr"-red] (photopsin I), green ["chlor"-green] (photopsin II), and bluish-violet light ["cyan"-bluish violet] (photopsin III). The violet cone pigment in the retina of the eye that was the first cone pigment studied chemically; also, a generic name for any cone pigment, though this sense is avoided in careful usage. Also called visual violet. [From iodine+Greek ops an eye+-ine indicating an organic compound, so called because the element iodine is violet in colour].

The next step is - Charge Stability is adding this concept to multiple Atoms. Size Matters. Charges have more stability on molecules than Atoms. When negative charges are associated with molecules they are delocalized.

Ok you probably need to go back and read the previous electrician manuals, this is like #8 or #9. We have covered quite a bit of ground that we can't fully recap, you need that information.

Induction - pulling electrons or pulling electron density, the action or process of inducting someone to a position or organization, the process of bringing on childbirth or abortion by artificial means, the production of an electric or magnetic state by the proximity (without contact) of an electrified or magnetized body, the production of an electric current in a conductor by varying the magnetic field applied to the conductor.

In molecules, stronger Adams will cause the electron density to "gravitate" towards them via induction. Remember that we said electricity is like water in previous manuals, and we jumped all the way out the window and said electricity is water in this one. My point is the Law of Maat always applies, balance is stability. Balance is stability but balance doesn't initiate reactions.

Alkyl Group - an alkyl group is an alkane missing one hydrogen.

Alkane -   of hydrogen and carbon atoms arranged

in a tree structure in which all the carbon–carbon bonds are single, compounds that consist entirely of single-bonded carbon and hydrogen atoms and lack any other functional groups.

Alkyls are important because they are electron donors, they are important similarly but opposite to electronegativity.

Alkaloids - any of a class of nitrogenous organic compounds of plant origin which have pronounced physiological actions on humans. They include many drugs (cocaine, morphine, quinine) and poisons (atropine, strychnine), **any of a class of naturally occurring organic nitrogen-containing <u>bases</u>**.

I made quite a few enemies in the Dr. Sebi family when I revealed that Mineral Elements, aren't the major medicinal or therapeutic compounds in plants. They had been selling their products based on the lie that they contained all the known minerals, which is 92 bwahahahahahaha...

Alkaloids are the major alkaline compounds in plants that have the most pronounced therapeutic effects, not the only though...

"When you breakdown our body, our biological

structure, into what we would have to put in it, chemistry, biochemistry. Melanin has no place, its not to be found in the body, that which is attributed to melanin is carbon" - Dr. Sebi

Oh don't forget the classic Dr. Sebi quote…

"Well white folks talk about protein. What is protein? They say one of the 19 amino acids, the building blocks of life… but I know for a fact that, that is not a true statement, because if protein was the building blocks of life, what happen to the gorilla that lives 180 years without eating anything that contains protein." - Dr. Sebi

I know, these ideas did not age well bwahahahahaha…

Amino Acids are tricky when you introduce the true idea of Acid-Base Reactions. Amino Acids are amphoteric, **they go both ways**. In fact how they function is completely dependent on their environment.

This is where the pKa becomes important, the pKa is the Meat number. The pKa tells you at what PH will half the molecules of a group be deprotonated, or at what PH will the number of deprotonated molecules match the number of protonated molecules. This allows you to predict Amino Acid behavior.

This is in our Osiris and Nepthys story, in the Osiris, Diabetes & Respiration book, please read &/or reread that book.

If the PH is lower than the pKa number, then you will have Acidic (Carboxylic Acid) behavior. If the PH is higher than the pKa number, then you will have Base/ Alkaline (Amine Group) behavior.

Titration - Titration is a common laboratory method

of quantitative chemical analysis to determine the concentration of an identified analyte (a substance whose chemical constituents are being identified and measured), the slow addition of one solution of a known concentration (called a titrant) to a known volume of another solution of unknown concentration until the reaction reaches neutralization, which is often indicated by a color change.

Titration is how you find out if you dealing with a Acidic or Alkaline substance, amongst other things...

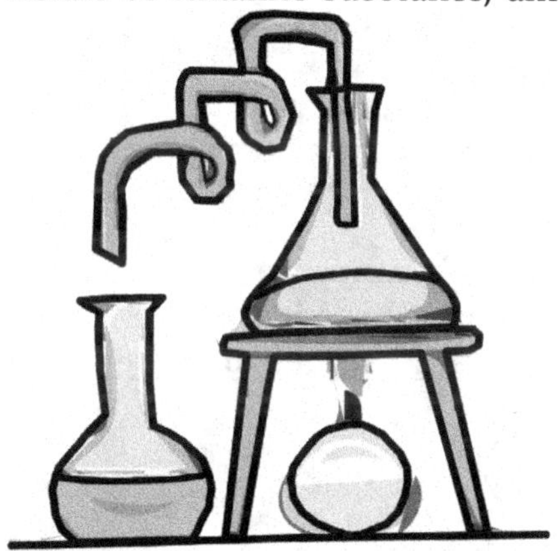

REDOX

The base of electrochemistry is the ability of chemical to produce electricity. What is our mantra?

Plasma carries electric currents, electric currents carry magnetic fields, alternating electric and magnetic fields produce light…

We have discussed this topic in maybe 30 of our 40+ books at this point but we have to do it again for clarity. **We are out here being cooked alive and no one seems to know or care**!

Redox is Electrochemistry!

Oxidation State - It describes the degree of oxidation (loss of electrons) of an atom in a chemical compound, the oxidation state may be positive, negative or zero, **the oxidation state of an atom is equal to the total number of electrons which have been removed from an element**.

Redox reactions can be created by applying a external voltage or by chemical reaction, hence the term electro/ chemistry.

Table Salt is a great example, when sodium reacts with chlorine, sodium donates an electron, creating an oxidation state of +1, chlorine accepts the electron so its oxidation state is reduced to −1.

Oxidation - Loss of Electrons

Reduction - Gain of Electrons

Reduction is binary, it takes two to tango. One atom or molecule is oxidizing or reducing another. When there are covalent bonds, the atom with the most electronegativity is said to have the electrons or cause induction. The electron donor is the reducing agent, or reductant, the electron acceptor is the oxidizing agent, or oxidant.

Electrochemical Cells use electrolytes to produce, conduct and transport electricity. Zinc is a popular Anode and Copper is a popular Cathode. Zinc readily losses electrons to Copper, sound familiar...?

Electrochemical Cell - a device that generates electrical energy from chemical reactions, splits the oxidant and reductant in a manner that allows electrons to flow through an external circuit from the reductant (which gets oxidized) to the oxidant (which causes reduction) while preventing them from physically touching each other.

Electrolyte - a charged mobile ion that functions as a conducting medium and in the case of "wet cells" is typically an aqueous solution of ionic compounds, a medium containing ions that are electrically conductive through the movement of those ions, but not conducting electrons, **substances that have a natural positive or negative electrical charge when dissolved in water**.

MELANOIDINS

Melanoidins - any of various brown, polymeric, often nitrogenous pigments formed when sugar and amino acids combine, brown, high molecular weight heterogeneous polymers that are formed when sugars and amino acids combine at high temperatures and low water activity, brown and flavorsome pigments found in malts and malt products. Melanoidins are formed when the reactive carbonyl group of the sugar reacts with the nucleophilic amino group of the amino acid. This process is accelerated in an alkaline environment, as the amino groups are deprotonated and, hence, have an increased nucleophilicity. WTF?!?!?!

Malt - barley or other grain that has been steeped, germinated, and dried, used for brewing or distilling and vinegar-making, convert (grain) into malt, prepared from cereal grain by allowing partial germination to modify the grain's natural food substances, to leave grain in water until it starts to grow, and then dry it to use in flour or in alcoholic drinks such as beer and whiskey (fermentation). Dextrose (corn sugar) and fructose (fruit sugar) are 100% fermentable by yeast, meaning the only calories left over are those from alcohol. Malt sugars, on the other hand, are only partially fermentable by yeast. These non-fermentable sugars are left over after fermentation and contribute additional calories.

I know that it is a large book but L'Goat book is a must read, please read &/or reread that book. In that book we discuss Osiris/Wusir have blood made from fermented fruit (grapes). In subsequent books like the PHD book etc.. we discuss the higher amount of type 2a fast twitch muscle brown and black people have. We have a built in mechanism of Fermentation to feed those muscle. Fermentation is preferred by cancer cells.

This is crazy!

You guys didn't understand the importance of me releasing the Beer & Bitters book! You still may not get it! The Bitters were the "cure" for the "Beer". Melanoidins are formed when the reactive carbonyl group of the sugar reacts with the nucleophilic amino group of the amino acid. This process is accelerated in an alkaline environment, as the amino groups are deprotonated and, hence, have an increased nucleophilicity.

A over alkaline diet will kill you!
Carbonyl Group - a carbonyl group is a functional group with the formula $C=O$, composed of a carbon atom double-bonded to an oxygen atom, a chemically organic functional group composed of a carbon atom double-bonded to an oxygen atom.

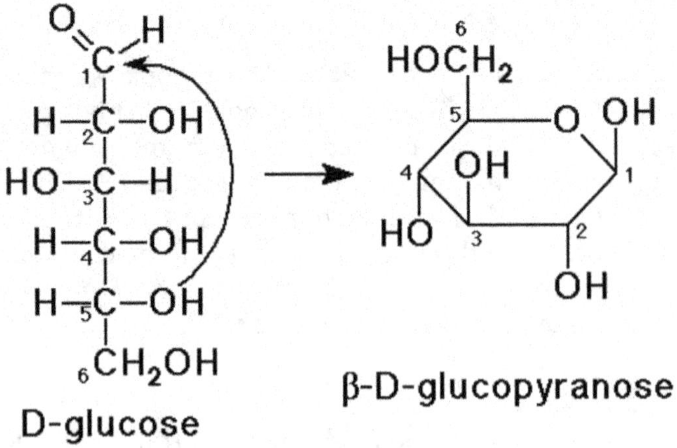

D-glucose → β-D-glucopyranose

Melanoidins are formed when the reactive carbonyl group of the sugar reacts with the nucleophilic amino group of the amino acid.

Anaerobic performances in black and white subjects

P F Ama 1, P Lagasse, C Bouchard, J A Simoneau
Affiliations expand

- PMID: 2402212

Abstract

The anaerobic performance characteristics of 15 Black males of African ancestry (25 +/- 2 yr; mean +/- SD) and 17 White males of French Canadian ancestry (22 +/- 2 yr) were compared. All subjects were sedentary. Morphological characteristics and body composition were similar in both groups. They were tested for maximal force during voluntary isometric contraction of the knee extensors and for total work output during 10 s, 30 s, and 90 s of maximal and repetitive knee extensions. Results indicated no significant differences between Blacks and Whites in maximal force of the knee extensors (736 +/- 78 N vs 722 +/- 11 N, respectively) and in total work output during the 10-s (1134 +/- 246 J vs 1124 +/- 207 J) and 30-s (2735 +/- 519 J vs 2779 +/- 647 J) tests. There was a difference of about 400 J between Blacks and Whites in the total work output during the 90-s test, but this difference was not statistically significant. However, significant differences were found between Blacks and Whites in the peak power output decrement during the last 60 s of the 90-s anaerobic test. These differences in peak power output between the two groups ranged between 7 and 10 W during the last 30 s of the 90-s test. The results indicate that knee extensor muscles of sedentary Black and White males have similar anaerobic performance power and capacities. However, **the results reveal that sedentary Black subjects experience a greater degree of fatigue than sedentary Whites during an anaerobic exercise lasting longer than 30 s**. This is a subtle but very dangerous thing to over look! After 30 seconds huh? We went into detail in Melanin vs Diabetes book 3 the Fiscal Edition & book 4 the Carbon Edition. We use the phosphates system initially, the first 9 seconds or so… The Clean Abs Fascia book maybe what you need to get the full picture but, **WE DON'T DO ANYTHING FOR UNDER 30 SECONDS IN REAL LIFE!**

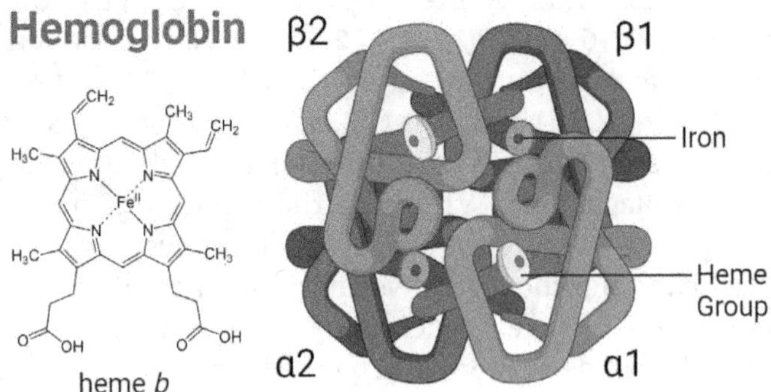

You guys didn't understand the importance of me releasing the Beer & Bitters book! You still may not get it! The Bitters were the "cure" for the "Beer". Melanoidins are formed when the reactive carbonyl group of the sugar reacts with the nucleophilic amino group of the amino acid. This process is accelerated in an alkaline environment, as the amino groups are deprotonated and, hence, have an increased nucleophilicity.

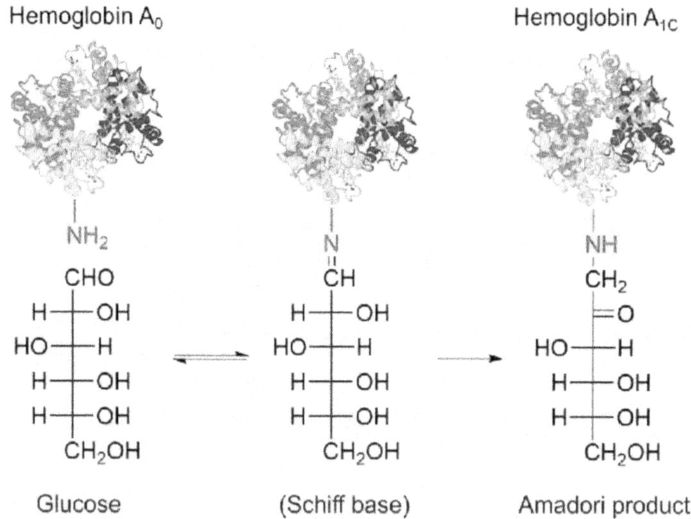
Hemoglobin A₀
Hemoglobin A₁C
NH₂
CHO
H OH
HO H
H OH
H OH
CH₂OH
Glucose
N
CH
H OH
HO H
H OH
H OH
CH₂OH
(Schiff base)
NH
CH₂
O
HO H
H OH
H OH
CH₂OH
Amadori product

Schiff Base - a vast group of compounds characterized by the presence of a double bond linking carbon and

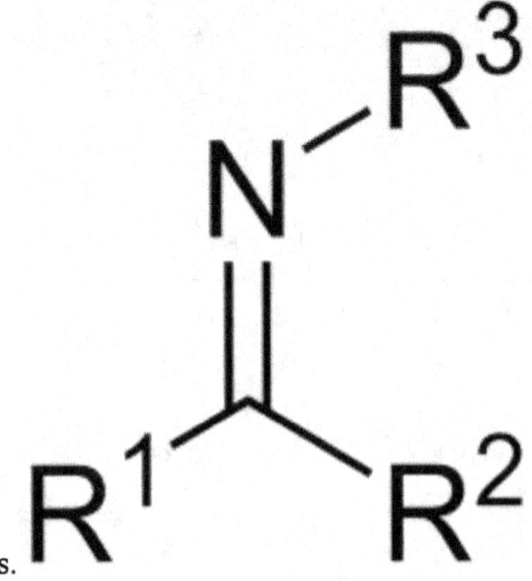

nitrogen atoms.

Amadori Products - Excess glucose can react with amino groups of intracellular and extracellular proteins in a nonenzymatic manner to form glycated residues termed as Amadori products, which subsequently undergo series of complex rearrangements yielding AGEs.

The Herbs in the Monthly Detox Kit at AmericanHealer.Website have been documented to help you break the bonds of Glycation!!! Follow the Blue Print in the Gold Book for specifics on how to apply this Science!

To get best results use the accountability system in the AlgaRhythm & Divine Mathematics Books.

"Well white folks talk about protein. What is protein?

They say one of the 19 amino acids, the building blocks of life... but I know for a fact that, that is not a true statement, because if protein was the building blocks of life, what happen to the gorilla that lives 180 years without eating anything that contains protein." - Dr. Sebi

If there was no such thing as protein then how was he "curing" diabetes? Bwahahahahaha

I have no doubt, that he was highly effective at fighting Diabetes, but whats sooooo funny, is **HE WAS CLUELESS**!

He got the instructions on what to do from a Mexican, but spoke about the black diet... LMMFAO... Why didn't he include Mexicans? Listen you guys have to relax out there! I love Sebi but we need scientific literacy, more than the free for all Herbal Salesmen!

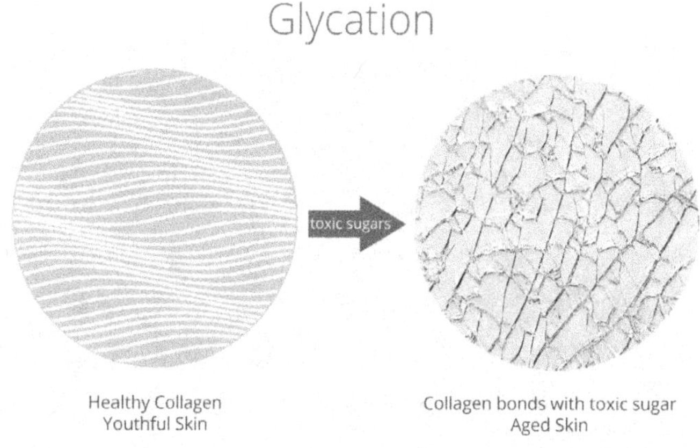

Your Fascia withers! Why? What do you think the Sugars hanging off your Blood Cells do? What have you learned

so far?

How effective can oxygen exchange be with a host of sugar molecules in the way?

Ok... We may need to shift gears, if water is the electricity and carrier of ions, proteins etc... The question may not be about the chemistry of Protein and Sugar, but Sugar Water...

.

SUGAR WATER

The bonds between oxygen and hydrogen, make the space near the oxygen negative and the space near the hydrogen positive. Water is not only a nucleophile but it's polar.

Similar to water, sucrose has bonds between oxygen and hydrogen
atoms, negative and positive. This makes the sugar very attractive (hydrophilic) via the areas of positive and negative charge. Carbon atoms play the background in the molecule, they don't contribute to sucrose being bipolar. You can see all the positive and negative charges though...

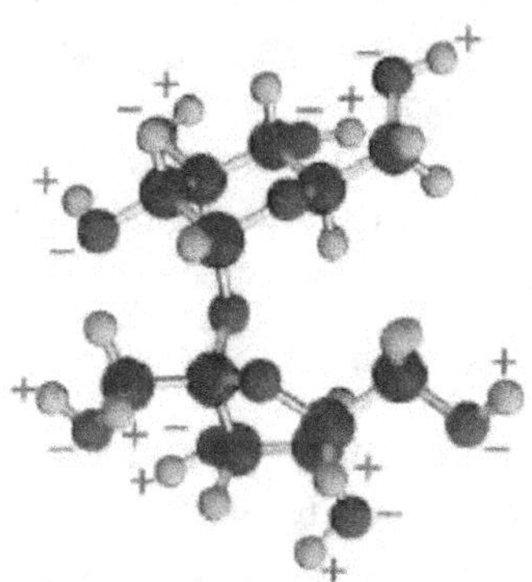

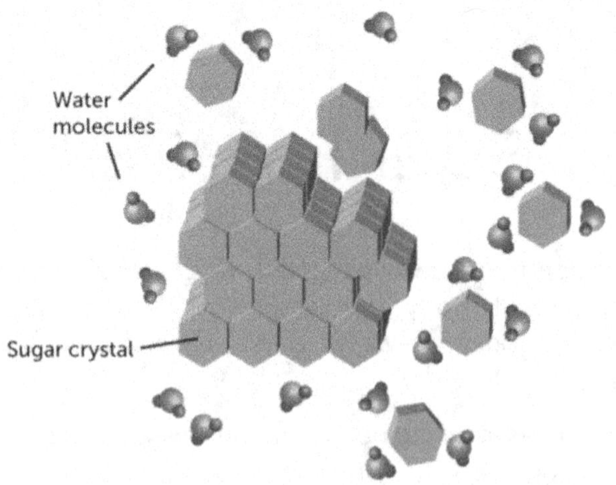

We have to really examine this from a few angles...
The more we can see what's going on, it may provide us with more insight. We have to fully understand this chemistry!!!

Adhesion - the action or process of adhering to a surface or object, the frictional grip of wheels, shoes, etc., on a road, track, or other surface, **the sticking together of particles of different substances**, an abnormal union of membranous surfaces due to inflammation or injury.
This is why we need to better understand that Light drives chemistry...

Heat Is ReaL Light...

Maybe we don't fully understand the nature of water! Hydrogen is Explosive & Oxygen is Fire, how do they combine and create Water? In water molecules Oxygen has a -2 oxidation state, that means it's highly stable. In water molecules Hydrogen has a +1 oxidation state, that means it is already oxidized! Oxidation is "burning" so in this sense the hydrogen is already burnt.

Oxidation…. Hmmmm… We may need to consider the idea that water is being changed from a Nucleophile, to an Electrophile. One of the most important qualities of water is it's nucleophilicity and its low viscosity. Sugar changes the nature of water. You know that Syrup is basically Sugar Water, you know the Honey is basically Sugar Water.

Sugar Water is clingy to everything, the nutrients in the blood get gluey. It's not just about oxygen! In the Was Sceptre book we discuss the 3,000+ proteins in the blood stream. Please go read &/or reread that book, think about the fly tape. Your blood cells are circulating with strands of fly tape on them! The viscosity levels go through the roof!

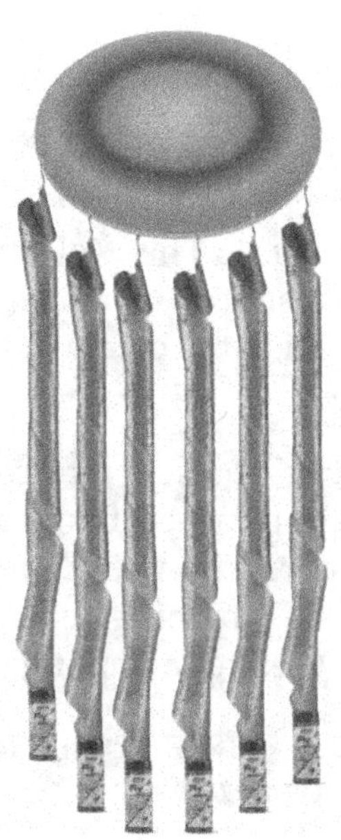

Bwahahahahaha... We have to open our minds chemically and think outside the box. Think about saturation.

Saturation - the state or process that occurs when no more of something can be absorbed, combined with, or added, the degree or extent to which something is dissolved or absorbed compared with the maximum possible, usually expressed as a percentage.

When Sugar reaches or surpassed the saturation ratio, it begins to become solid in the liquid! That's how Syrup & Honey have that thickness. The ratio for sugar and water 2:1, 14 pints of sugar in 7 pints of water (plasma).

We go into culinary school from there! Adjusting body heat aka temperature is a sure fire way to attempt to control chemistry. Hot Flashes, Fevers, Cold Sweats, B3 Heat/Itch.... are all apart of self regulation!

Le Châtlier's Principle - A change in one of the variables that describe a system at equilibrium produces a shift in the position of the equilibrium that counteracts the effect of this change.

The Maillard reaction - The Maillard reaction is an organic chemical reaction in which reducing sugars react with amino acids to form a complex mixture of compounds.

Glycation—sometimes also referred to as non-enzymatic glycosylation—occurs during the initial stage of the Maillard reaction, the first step in a complex series of Maillard or browning reactions that proceed spontaneously between reducing sugars and proteins.

Excessive urine is a defense mechanism, it's a way to pull off sugar. We have too much sugar, we are over saturated with sugar and insulin! We are going to get dehydrated, if we don't get more ion, fiber rich water into our bodies quickly! Equatorial Haplotypes are supposed to not only be consuming fiber and pigment with their sugars but also **CITRIC ACID**! Drops the PH, slows reverses glycation and crystallization of sugar!

When you eat, you break zillions of bonds. Breaking all the bonds of your food and producing all those enzymes takes energy, cools the system a bit. This pushes the system to balance the system, boost temperature back up. Le Châtlier's Principle cause more glycation. We need energy, but because the blood is getting coated with sugar reparation is less efficient.

When we exercise the sugar doesn't have a chance to make candy out of our Red Blood Cells. Think about the boiling point, 212 degrees, that's an approximation. The boiling point is actually whenever vapor pressure equals atmospheric pressure. I think we have a similar process going on when we begin to dilate blood vessels and sweat to reduce heat. Skeletal muscles working pushes the body temperature up, it keeps sugar dissolved until it can be digested. The faster the muscles contract and relax, the higher the internal temperature, the more sugar you can tolerate. When the body is cooling that sugar recrystallizes into candy!!! If you don't exercise forget about it!!!

Dr. Sebi did not promote exercise, there is no one anywhere that can show you a clip of Dr. Sebi promoting exercise because he did not understand chemistry. He believed protein was imaginary…

Syrups and candies are made simply by heating water, heating water allows the water to hold more than a 2 to 1 ratio. When you turn off the heat the sugar that is not bound by the water molecules bonds back to each other, not to mention the fact you lose water in the boiling process. In your blood that process has a drain, the tricarboxylic acid cycle or the citric acid cycle. The sugar is supposed to be pulled out of the circulation by hungry muscles!!!

The Myoglobin in the skeletal muscles has a higher oxygen affinity, this drains the blood. At least in a working system it does.

Glycation = Crystallization based on Le Châtelier's principle: a system that is shifted away from equilibrium acts to restore equilibrium by reacting in opposition to the shift.

Digestion of carbohydrates without a demand for them via exercise puts a strain on the system. Increase in body heat causes the system to decrease energy a regular aspect of "Naggeritis" in an attempt to bring the body heat and energy expenditure down. The break down of chemical bonds in carbohydrates always absorbs energy, cooling the system down, so more sugar molecules dissolve in the plasma.

Glycation. Which is also explained by Le Châtelier's principle: You just go straight to sleep uncontrollably or get tired and cranky! It's a decrease in body heat causing the system to generate energy, in an attempt to restore the body heat.

We discussed the endothermic vs exothermic reaction of forming and breaking bonds.

The creation of chemical bonds always releases energy (out of the body), more sugar molecules join glycation in an attempt to increase the body heat. This is why glycation happens when the body heat decreases.

Glycation changes all of the redox reactions that happen in healthy clean blood. Here is a way to remember this stuff every time you see the word Glycation.

Cation - a positively charged ion, i.e. one that would be attracted to the cathode in electrolysis.
Glyco - Sugar

Glycol + Cation = GlyCation, remember those positive ions as oxidants or free radicals in this context. These changes to cellular geometry, turbulence and fluid dynamics, lead to high blood pressure as well as clogged lymph nodes. You might as well forget about clogged arteries, you are creating clogged lymph vessels and lymph nodes. The receptor for advanced glycation end-products (RAGE) is a newly recognized factor regulating cancer cell invasion and metastasis. Why do you think thyroid hormone replacement is associated with a decrease in A1C level? Iodine is big and electron hungry!

Evidence for the role of lipid peroxides on glycation of hemoglobin and plasma proteins in non-diabetic asthma patients

V Sathiyapriya 1, Zachariah Bobby, S Vinod Kumar, N Selvaraj, V Parthibane, Swapnil Gupta
Affiliations expand

- PMID: 16380104 DOI: 10.1016/j.cca.2005.11.001

Abstract

Background: Collective evidences reveal that malondialdehyde (MDA), reduced glutathione (GSH) and ascorbic acid can modulate protein glycation. We investigated the concentrations of MDA, GSH, ascorbic acid and protein glycation in asthma patients to delineate the possible association among these parameters.

Methods: Blood was collected from 18 asthma patients and 16 age and sex matched control subjects. Glycated hemoglobin (HbA1C), GSH, MDA, vitamin C, fructosamine and glucose were assessed in both groups. The effect of H2O2 on glycation of hemoglobin was studied by incubating normal healthy erythrocytes with either 5 or 50 mmol/l glucose concentration.

Results: Plasma of asthma patients revealed significantly higher concentrations of lipid peroxides and fructosamine concentrations than the matched controls. Glycated hemoglobin concentrations were also found to be significantly increased. Ascorbic acid and GSH concentrations were decreased significantly in the test group when compared with the healthy control group. When the effects of fasting glucose, GSH and ascorbic acid on the concentrations of HbA1C and fructosamine were refuted by partial correlation analysis, MDA was found to be a significant determinant of HbA1c and fructosamine in patients with asthma. The in vitro model with human erythrocytes showed an enhancement of protein glycation by H2O2.

Conclusion: An increased glycation of proteins was found in asthma patients. These data also support the premise that lipid peroxides per se do have a role to play in glycation of hemoglobin and plasma proteins.

Yes H2O2 (Set) plays a major role in this process, **GLYCATION INHIBITS CATALASE REACTIONS**!!! BLOCKING ELECTROCHEMISTRY IS THE ESSENCE OF DIABETES!!!

We now have a new vocabulary word, glycation =

corrosion.

Corrosion - a natural process that converts a refined metal into a more chemically stable oxide, occurs when most or all of the atoms on the same metal surface are oxidized, damaging the entire surface, as the degradation of a metal due to a reaction with its environment.

Glycation - a natural process that converts a refined pigment into a more chemically stable oxide, occurs when most or all of the atoms on the same pigment surface are oxidized, damaging the entire surface, as the degradation of a pigment due to a reaction with its environment.

Why do you think our kidneys are failing? Please read &/or reread EnQi & the Brain Wave book, we detail the kidney chemistry. The liver is the chief site of ammonia detoxication, of the liberation of glucose, and of urea formation.

Do you understand so far?

Ammonia metabolism in exercise and fatigue: a review

B J Mutch, E W Banister
·   PMID: 6341752

Abstract

Although fatigue is a well-known phenomenon and the phrase "exercised until exhaustion" is commonly understood, there is no unequivocal agreement on **the fundamental nature of the fatigue process**. Ammonia was linked to the development of fatigue as early as 1922, when ammonia production was observed from stimulated nerve and the question whether there could be a relationship between **ammonia production and the muscle activity** was raised. The immediate source of ammonia from muscle appears to be a result of the **deamination of AMP and is more apparent in fast-twitch than in slow-twitch fibers.** More recently, increases in blood ammonia levels have been reported in rats after swimming and in humans after arm work, maximal cycle ergometry, and treadmill exercise. Elevated blood ammonia has also been linked to a surprising variety of functional and metabolic neurological disturbances other than exercise and fatigue, including the development of hepatic coma, convulsions from ammonia toxicity precipitated by high-pressure oxygen breathing, epileptic seizures, and decreased neuronal excitability. In addition, a number of genetic disorders (inborn errors in metabolism, or IEMs) are characterized by elevated blood ammonia concentrations. Symptoms of neural disability in all of the above conditions have been related to the concentration of ammonia in blood. Although these studies do not relate to exercise or fatigue directly, it is conceivable that our understanding of the effect of high concentrations of blood ammonia in these clinical conditions may provide valuable insight into the effect of ammonia during exercise. This paper reviews the effect of ammonia production during exercise and other conditions upon purposeful activity and the development of fatigued states.

To be continued lol

Ammonia and Water are the basic nucleophiles of biochemistry. Ammonia and Water up regulate the conductivity of melanin, the Holy Grail of Melanin Properties.

Evolving on a high carbohydrate diet, Equatorial People use muscle activity, for circulation, digestion and ammonia metabolism into urea. Exercise takes the strain off the Kidneys & Liver, directly under fire by glycation. Exercise and Herbs...

The Herbs are at AmericanHealer.Website

The Books are on Amazon

The Power is in your hands now!

Let me link these for you...

ATP becomes ADP becomes AMP... That means the tank is empty, AMPK is the sensor to refill the tank... Get it? AMPK works with MCH to kick in Autophagy...

Autophagy destroys Glycation...

You don't have to starve your way into Autophagy, the Bitters we have, the Monthly Detox Kit and the exercises we lay out in the Gold Book all initiate and accelerate Autophagy! Safely!

History of Bioelectrical Study and the Electrophysiology of the Primo Vascular System

Sang Hyun Park, 1 Eung Hwi Kim, 1 Ho Jong Chang, 1 Seung Zhoo Yoon, 2 Ji Woong Yoon, 3 Seong-Jin Cho, 4 and Yeon-Hee Ryu 4 , 5 ,* Author information Article notes Copyright and License information PMC Disclaimer

Go to:

Abstract

Background. Primo vascular system is a new anatomical structure whose research results have reported the possibility of a new circulatory system similar to the blood vascular system and cells. Electrophysiology, which measures and analyzes bioelectrical signals tissues and cells, is an important research area for investigating the function of tissues and cells. The bioelectrical study of the primo vascular system has been reported by using modern techniques since the early 1960s by Bonghan Kim. This paper reviews the research result of the electrophysiological study of the primo vascular system for the discussion of the circulatory function. We hope it would help to study the electrophysiology of the primo vascular system for researchers. This paper will use the following exchangeable expressions: Kyungrak system = Bonghan system = Bonghan circulatory system = primo vascular system = primo system; Bonghan corpuscle = primo node; Bonghan duct = primo vessel. We think that objective descriptions of reviewed papers are more important than unified expressions when citing the papers. That said, this paper will unify the expressions of the primo vascular system.

Go to:

1. Primo Vascular System

The primo vascular system has been studied as part of the anatomical and histological research of the last 10 years. It is a novel thread-like structure that remains unrevealed in animals and humans. Particularly, the primo vascular system was selected as the feature article and for the cover page in the Journal of Anatomical Record [1]; it provoked controversy in the anatomical society and among acupuncture scientists. Since then, the discovery of the primo vascular system in lymphatic vessels [2], cardiac vascular vessels [3], and the brain [4] has received much attention.

Early scientists of the primo vascular system, who focused on anatomical and histological studies, hypothesized about the relationship between oriental medicine and acupuncture and the meridian. These findings are helping to integrate the theories of conventional and alternative medicine [5].

Kim, who initially studied the anatomical structures of the acupuncture and the meridian, declared that "This project developed from our inherited oriental medicine, which is our ancestors' creative and noble endeavor as approved at the third Joseon Labor Party Congress" in his first paper [6].

Moreover, Soh considered that Bonghan corpuscles and ducts were identical to acupuncture sites and meridians [5], stating his theory that the Bonghan circulatory system may be an extension of acupuncture and meridians [7]. It was reported that DNA was in the primo vascular system [1]; evidence showing that the primo vascular system may be a DNA circulatory system has been reported as well [4].

Electrophysiology is a science of the electrical properties of biological tissues and cells. It involves measurements of voltage changes or electric current on a wide variety of scales from single-ion channel proteins to whole organs such as the heart. In this paper, we introduce the history of electrical signals and the electrophysiology of the primo vascular system.

Section 2 introduces the understanding of electrophysiology and modern techniques to measure the bioelectrical signal for general readers. Section 3 describes the beginning of the bioelectrical study of acupuncture meridian briefly and reviews the electrophysiological study of the primo vascular system past and present. The last section arranges the result of the reviewed papers and suggests the future work for the electrophysiology of the primo vascular system.

Go to:

2. Development of Electrophysiology with Electrical Signal and Basic Medicine

2.1. Bioelectrical Signal Studies and Electrophysiology

In 1791, the Italian physician and physicist Luigi Galvani first recorded the phenomenon of electrical signals while dissecting a frog on a table where he had been conducting experiments with static electricity (Figure 1). Galvani coined the term animal electricity to describe the phenomenon, while contemporaries labeled it galvanism. Galvani and his contemporaries regarded muscle activation as resulting from an electrical fluid or substance in the nerves [8, 9].

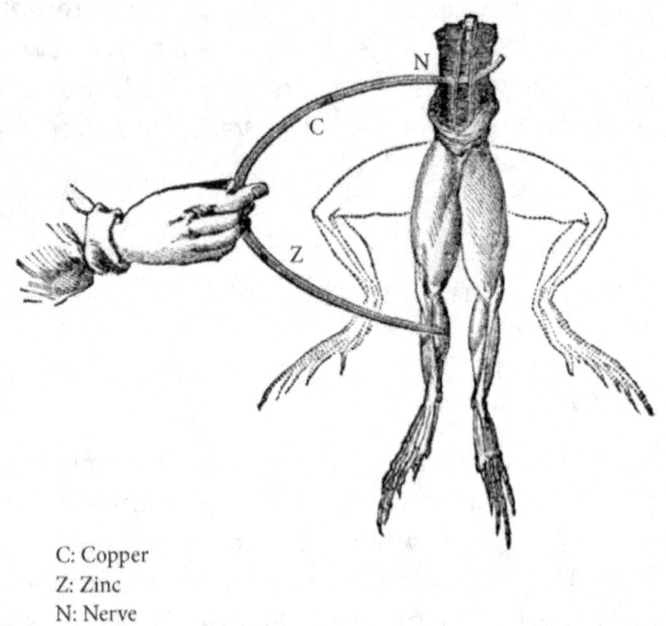

C: Copper
Z: Zinc
N: Nerve

Figure 1

The electrical stimulation of a frog nerve. It was found that the current flows through the two different metals, coming into contact with animal muscle.

In the work to study cardiac electrophysiology in order to gain a better understanding of bioelectricity, cardiac electrophysiology emerged as an important area to elucidate and diagnose the heart function and to treat heart disease, including arrhythmia, through electrocardiograms (Figure 2) [10]. The function of tissues and organs in humans is closely related to analyses of the bioelectrical signals from these features.

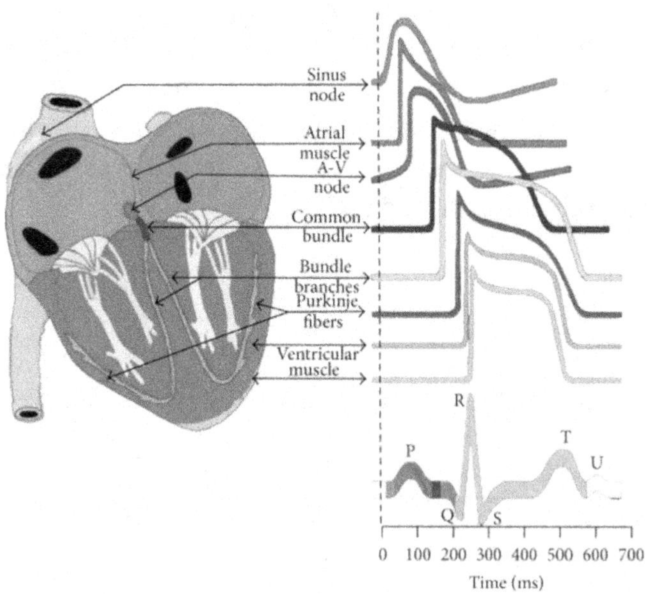

Figure 2

Electrophysiology of the heart.

2.2. Development of a Measurement Method for Bioelectric Signals

Electrophysiological studies, which started from frog muscle response research, extended the fundamental knowledge of nerve cells through squid axon membrane potential measurements using an electrode when Hodgkin and Huxley began this work in 1952 [11]. Graham and Gerard succeeded to create and develop an electrode with a finer diameter of 2–5 um to measure the intracellular potential (Figure 3) [12]. With the development of this measurement technique, Neher and Sakmann reduced the signal-to-noise ratio using a seamless seal between the cell membrane and the electrode, establishing the foundation of the study of ion channels in the cell membrane [13]. Cell membrane potential measurement techniques in electrophysiological research are outlined later.

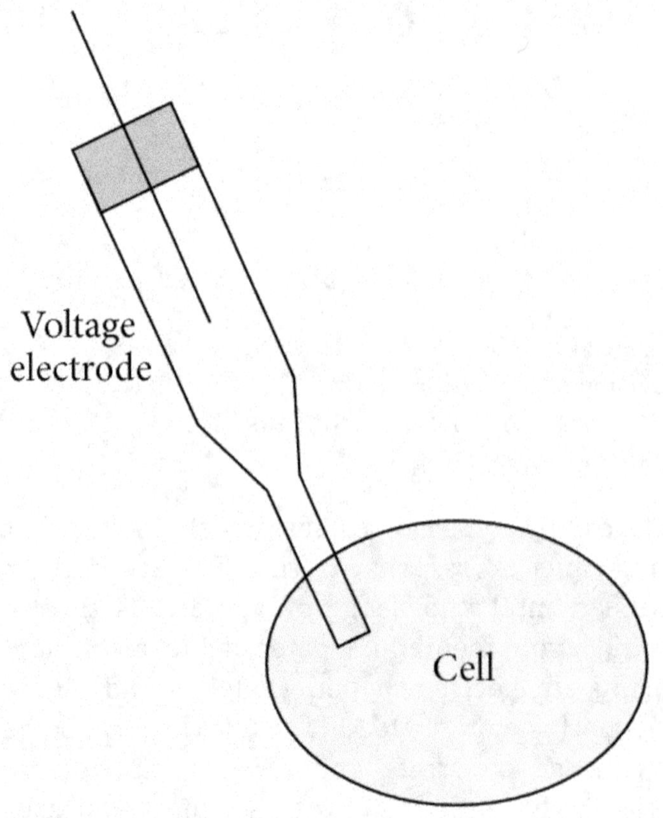

Figure 3
Intracellular recording technique.

2.2.1. Intracellular Recording (Voltage Clamp and

Current Clamp)

An electrical signal representing cell activities is a result of the activity of the ion channels in the cell membrane. The cell activity is associated with whether the cell membrane ion channel is activating or not and is then related to the electrical signals from the cells. Related to this, the voltage clamp technique was developed to measure the intracellular ion flow with the constant membrane potential. This technique was useful in research on the mechanism of biological electrical signals generated by the ions such as K + or Na+ passing through the electrically opened and closed channels [11–13].

In contrast, the current clamp was used to measure the changes of the voltage inside the cell by means of a constant current; this was useful to classify cell types by understanding the action potential of the cells (**Figure 4**) [14, 15].

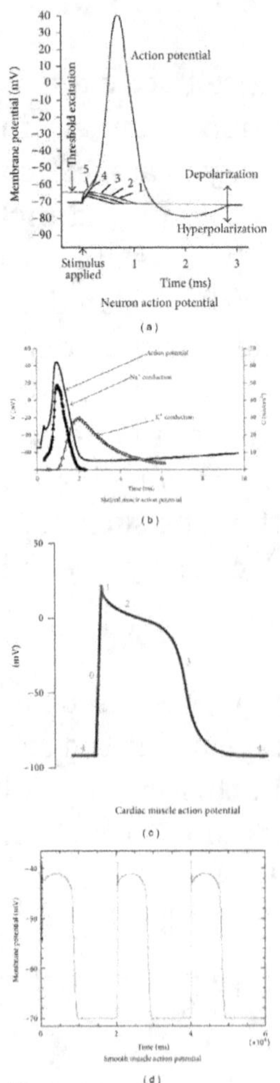

Figure 4

A comparison of the action potentials of major tissue cells.

2.2.2. Patch Clamp

As an intracellular recording technique which involves inserting an electrode into a cell directly, the patch clamp technique was created for the purpose of separating and analyzing of each ion channel existing on the membrane of a cell. Patch clamp recordings use, as an electrode, a glass micropipette that has an open tip diameter of about one micrometer (1 μm), which is a size enclosing a membrane surface area or "patch" that often contains just one or few ion channel molecules. This type of electrode is distinct from the "sharp microelectrode" used to impale cells in traditional intracellular recordings, in that it is sealed onto the surface of the cell membrane rather than inserted through it. Many researchers, including Neher and Sakmann, studied ion channels in various cells using the patch clamp technique (Figure 5) [16–18].

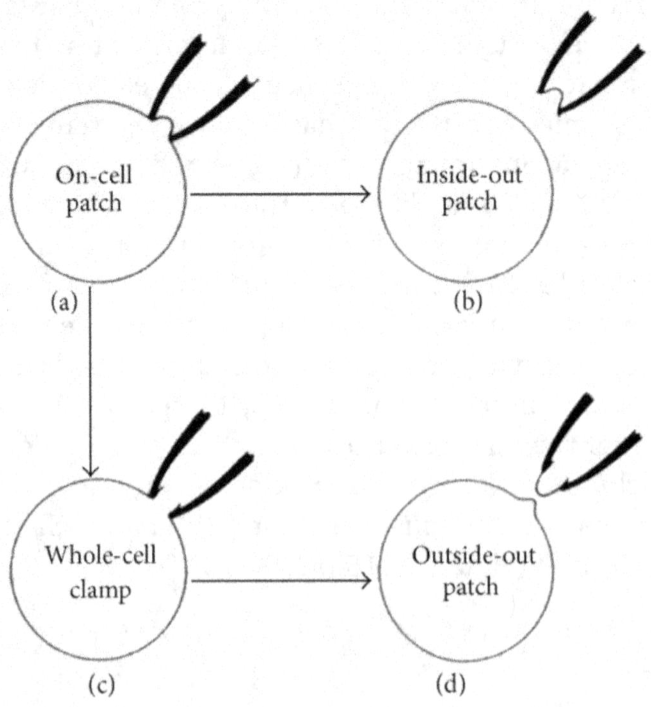

Figure 5

Patch clamp technique.

They observed that the electrophysiological characteristics in each major tissue cell, especially the resting potential, showed a different form (Table 1). This cell-size level technique led to the development of electrophysiology and has produced many eminent scientists and Nobel Award winners [19–22].

Table 1

A comparison of electrophysiological characteristics between tissues.

	Neur on	Muscle		
		Skelet al	Cardiac	Smooth
Resting potential (mV)	-70	-80 to -90	-85 to -95	-50 to -60
Threshold potential (mV)	-55	-55	Spike potentia l	Spike potentia l
Action potential duration (ms)	1	2 to 5	200 to 400	10 to 50

Open in a separate window

The development of the measurement technique such as intracellular recording and patch clamp advanced the electrophysiological research.

Go to:

3. Beginning of Electrophysiology of the Primo Vascular System

Although the primo vascular system has been studied intensively over last 10 years, there is no complete evidence of whether the primo vascular system is an extension of acupuncture and meridians system or is identical to acupuncture and meridians, which are key concepts in oriental medicine. Oriental medicine scientists scarcely accept hypotheses pertaining to the anatomical structures of acupuncture and meridians. However, in their work on the primo vascular system, Soh [7] and Lee et al. [23] declared that they were inspired by Bonghan Kim's theory from the 1960s [6, 24–27]. Therefore, the beginning of the electrophysiology of the primo vascular system established a standard from the beginning of the measurement of the electrical properties related to acupuncture and meridians.

3.1. Historical Trends of the Bioelectrical Study of Acupuncture and Meridians

The bioelectrical signal measurements of acupuncture and meridians were attempts to determine the existence of these structures. These studies were done using animals and cadavers; it was assumed that human study was only partially complete.

Jeh found that acupuncture points had lower resistance than the surrounding skin by measuring the skin resistance [28]. Overhof verified that the resistance at acupuncture points was lower than that of nonacupuncture points [29]. Later, Ogata et al. reported that acupuncture points had lower resistance than non-acupuncture points located in the same meridian [30]. In particular, Niboyet's methods have led to the development of ear acupuncture, which has become one of the acupuncture treatment therapies offered in Europe. Considering this low-resistance feature, Voll designed an acupuncture diagnostic apparatus using microcurrents [31].

Studies of the low-resistance properties of acupuncture points have been performed intermittently. Recently, Ahn et al. took ultrasonic images of acupuncture points and proposed, anatomically, that a collagenous band in connective tissues was related to the low-impedance property of acupuncture points [32].

A modern system to be able to measure the resistance of acupuncture point has been developed recently based on the result of the lower resistance on the acupoint [33].

But there are still limitations to measure the special point on the skin by classical theory and method since 1950s.

3.2. Bioelectrical Study and Electrophysiology of the Primo Vascular System in the 1960s

Kim published five papers in total about the existence of the anatomical structure of meridians at the Kyungrak Institute in the 1960s [6, 24–27, 34]. Three out of the five papers described electrical signal measurements and analyses of acupuncture points and meridians. His first paper investigated the electrical properties of acupuncture points and meridians. The following description was extracted from his first paper, given at the conference of the Pyongyang Medical School on October 18, 1961:

"This project was started to develop and propagate oriental medicine, which is our ancestor's creative and noble endeavor as approved at the third Joseon Labor Party Congress... We have set ourselves an assignment to find the electrical properties of meridians first and then the Kyungrak system based on these properties" [6].

Kim already knew about research reports on the electrical resistance of acupuncture points, showing that it was lower than the areas around the spots. He had attempted to measure and examine unseen singular points on the skin. When writing his paper, he investigated the electrical properties of acupuncture by measuring the resistance and voltage around the acupuncture points of rabbits. The resistance value was about 20,000–80,000 Ω when applying 100 μA, and it was lower than the values around the point. He indicated the problem of the changing measurement value in terms of the measurement time, interval, and number of measurements. However, the locations of the low-resistance points were fixed; the distribution of the locations coincided with the acupuncture points described in the Dongui Bogam, which is a physician Book of

Traditional Medicine compiled by Heo Jun in 1613 during the Joseon Dynasty of Korea [35].

It was surprising that he had found that the voltage value of the acupuncture point changed consistently. The voltage change was a regular and rhythmical wave group with a wave period of 3–6 sec and an intensity level of 0.1 mV. He reported that 5–7 waves were detected continuously, followed by a resting phase (**Figure 6**). He asserted that non-acupuncture points did not display this phenomenon (**Figure 7**).

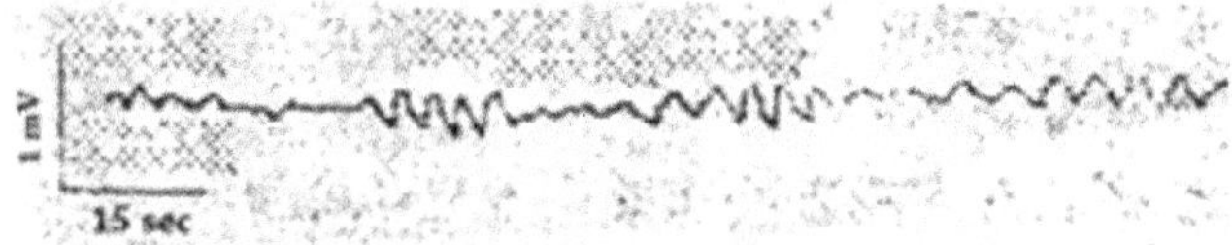

Figure 6
The electric induction on a Nogung acupuncture point (PC8).

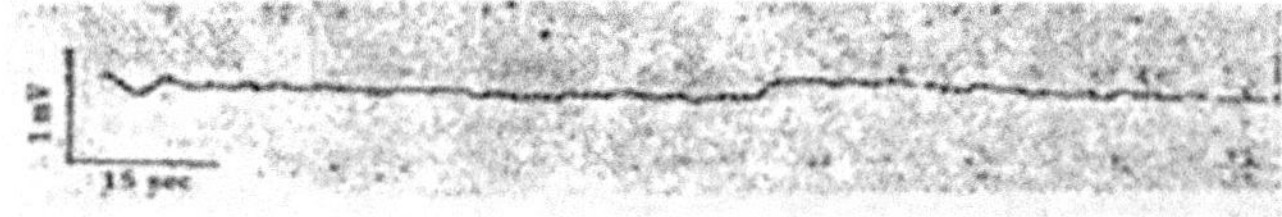

Figure 7
The induced electricity at non-acupuncture points located 1 cm from Nogung.

He considered that the changing values of acupuncture points may be connected to physiological properties and therefore ran an interrelationship experiment.

It was an experiment to measure the interactional electrical signals between stimulation by a needle and large intestine movements. He reported some interaction between acupoint ST36 and the movement of the large intestine when measuring the electrical signals and stimulating the intestine (Figure 8).

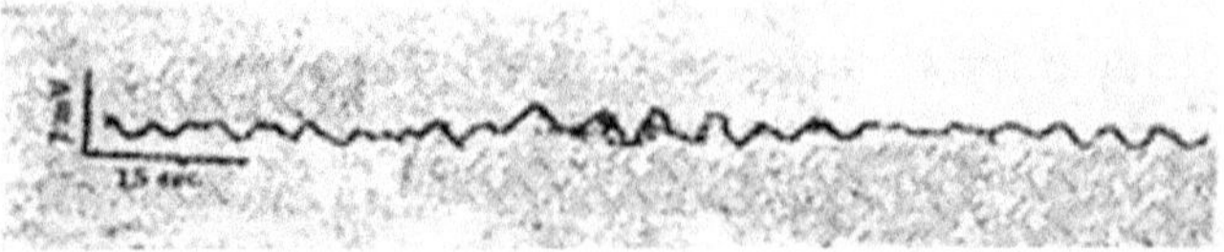

Figure 8
The induced electricity at an acupuncture point after hyperkinesis of the large intestine.

His interpretation of the result from his interaction experiment was different from those of general acupuncture scientists at that time. He suggested that acupuncture and internal organs should be connected materially to each other, hypothesized that acupuncture points and meridians would be anatomical structures in the human body, and started to explore anatomical tissues (Figure 9).

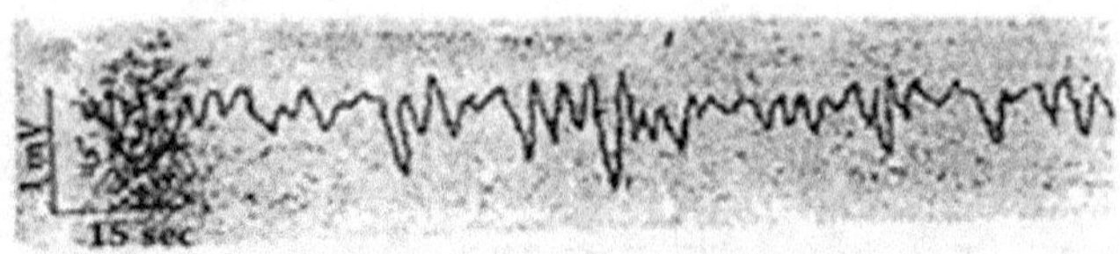

Figure 9
The electric induction on the Susamni acupuncture point

(LI10).

B. H. Kim advanced anatomical and histological research and Kyungrak circulatory research by developing his first paper into his second published paper, entitled On the Acupuncture Meridian System.

He named the discovered anatomical structures around acupuncture points Bonghan corpuscles and the thread-like structure connected to Bonghan corpuscles Bonghan ducts. (He did not use the word Bonghan system. He only named the new anatomical and histological structures of Kyungrak system Bonghan corpuscles and Bonghan ducts [24].)

In order to investigate the circulation of the Kyungrak system, he analyzed the physiological and bioelectrical measurements of Bonghan corpuscles first, as this was the basis of the contention that the morphological characteristics of Bonghan corpuscles were smooth muscles and secreting cells.

He inserted an electrode directly into a Bonghan corpuscle and measured the bioelectrical signal from Bonghan corpuscle. It was very similar to the extracelluar recording method in the modern technical term. But there were limitations to be able to measure the bioelectrical signal from the tissue of Bonghan corpuscle because of noises. Now modern technique to measure the bioelectrical signal can measure the electrical signal from single cells [36].

The physiological study of Bonghan corpuscles and ducts progressed as the manner in which bioelectrical signals changed by various stimulations was studied.

He proposed that Bonghan corpuscles and ducts responded to various stimuli and that the responses were similar to those of nerves. There were many experiments conducted to determine where the signal was conducted—whether it was along the Bonghan corpuscle and duct or another area [6].

The bioelectrical research into Bonghan corpuscles recorded the changing values of the bioelectrical signals by inserting an electrode into a Bonghan corpuscle. The experimental result reported that the change of the potential in a Bonghan corpuscle was similar to a sine curve, terming this curve a "" (geu) wave with a period of 3–6 seconds. Also identified was a "" (neu) wave at 7–10 seconds and a "" (deu) wave at 20–25 seconds. The amplitude of each wave was 0.1 mV (Figure 10).

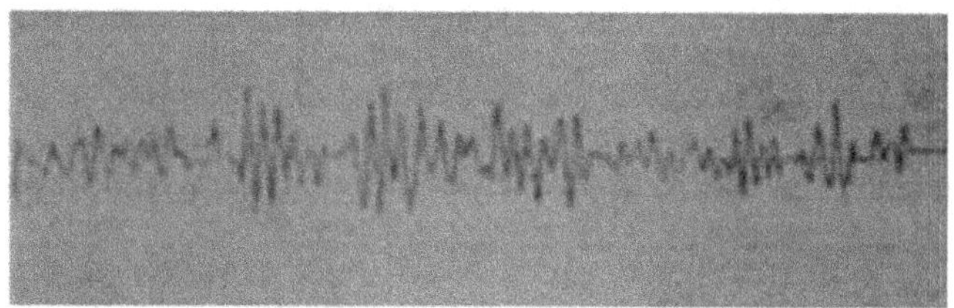

Figure 10

The bioelectrical activity from a Bonghan corpuscle.

Particularly, these electric potential changes disappeared when the temperature of the environment dropped below 27°C but reappeared when the temperature was raised to 39°C immediately. He suggested that the bioelectrical properties of acupuncture points as explained by the nervous system were incorrect, as the phenomena of the changing signal appeared from Bonghan corpuscles, which are not related to the nervous system.

The next experiment involved assessing the excitability and response of Bonghan corpuscle by various stimuli. B. H. Kim expressed that *"the study of excitability of Bonghan corpuscles was a basic problem to elucidate the physiological functions of the Kyungrak system."* Acetylcholine and pilocarpine were used and the electrical potential changes were recorded.

The experiment result reported that the bioelectrical signals changed after stimulation with acetylcholine, pilocarpine, and Novocain.

He noted that the signals varied according to the different types and concentration of drugs (Figure 11). Finally, the experiment of the bioelectrical signal conduction of the Kyungrak system was based on his first paper, which reported the interaction materially and functionally between Bonghan corpuscles and internal organs (Figure 12) [6]. This study was significant in that it determined how the stimulation signals of Bonghan corpuscles were delivered in the Kyungrak system. He stimulated Bonghan corpuscles connected to a Bonghan duct to measure the bioelectrical potential of the next Bonghan corpuscle. The experimental result reported that the bioelectrical potential changed after a certain time and that the delivery speed of the effect stimuli was 3.0 mm/sec at a superficial Bonghan corpuscle (a Bonghan corpuscle in the skin).

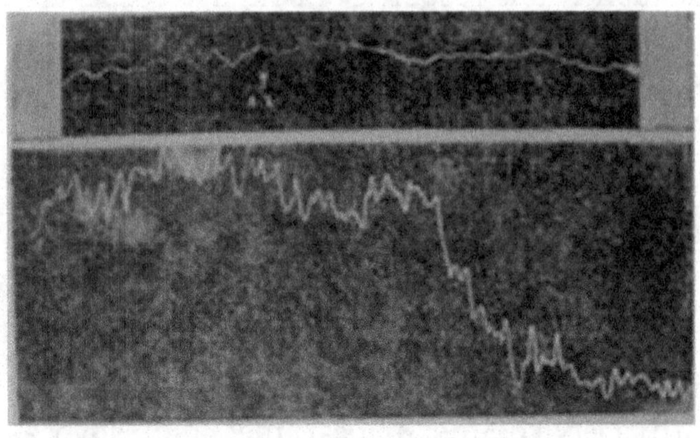

Figure 11
The changes in the bioelectrical activity of a Bonghan corpuscle after an injection of acetylcholine.

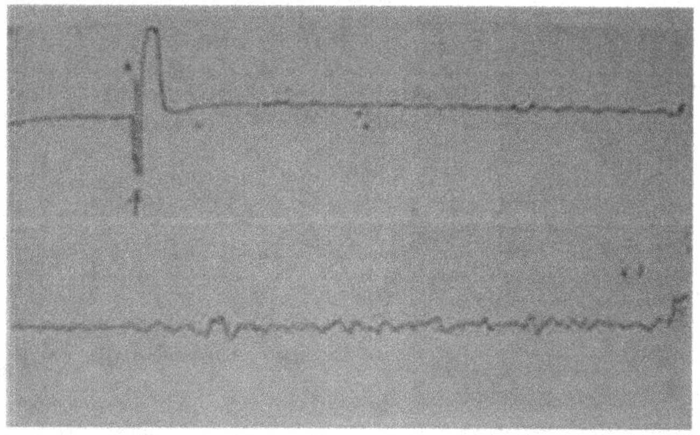

Figure 12
Strong electrical stimulation amplifies the changes in the bioelectrical activity of a Bonghan corpuscle.

The relationship between mechanical movements and the bioelectrical signals of Bonghan ducts was reported in his third paper. It started with an exploration of Bonghan ducts, not Bonghan corpuscles, and developed this line of research from previous results. The properties of bioelectrical signals were similar to those of a superficial Bonghan corpuscle (a Bonghan corpuscle in the skin), and the delivery speed was 1–3 mm/sec for communication in both directions. He asserted that the phenomena of longitudinal periodic lateral and pulsatory mixed movement could be observed [25]. The movement delivery speed of the Bonghan duct was 0.1–0.6 mm/sec, which was much slower than that of the bioelectrical signals. However, the experimental results pertaining to the relationship between the mechanical movement and bioelectrical changing were limited because the explanation of the experiment setup and data was insufficient. Nonetheless, he insisted that there was convincing evidence of the flow of liquid actively through Bonghan ducts. Afterward, his study concentrated on Sanal cells (primo microcells) and the liquid through Bonghan ducts.

Go to:

4. Recent Bioelectrical and Electrophysiology Research on the Primo Vascular System

Electrophysiological research on the primo vascular system halted after his third paper. His fourth and fifth papers were focused on flowing Bonghan liquids and Sanal cells through Bonghan corpuscles and ducts. Park started to measure and analyze the electrical potential of Bonghan corpuscles in the 2000s (Figure 13) [37]. Various experiments involving the staining Bonghan corpuscles and ducts were attempted to distinguish them from other tissues [4, 23, 38–42]. Lee et al. reported that trypan blue was the most effective type of stain for these corpuscles and ducts in 2007 [4]. The trypan blue staining method was advanced by B. C. Lee. Park attempted to stain Bonghan corpuscles using the trypan blue staining method and attempted to measure and analyze the electrical signals from Bonghan corpuscles of the intestines of rats [37]. He worked on three main research topics, measuring and analyzing the resting potential and spontaneous action potential using an intracellular recording method. He also observed the changing electrical potential by stimulation with various drugs, such as acetylcholine, modeled the electrical signals by BVP (Bonhoeffer-Van der Pol) modeling, and analyzed the findings by fractal theory. J. H. Choi, C. J. Choi, and Cho developed the electrophysiology of the primo vascular system after this research [43–45].

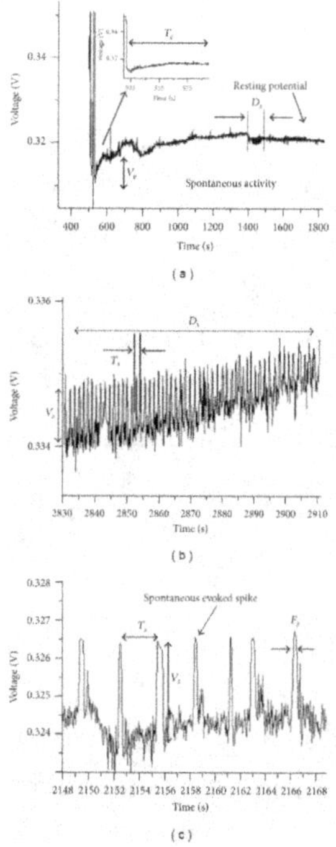

Figure 13

Resting potential and spontaneous activity of the potential in a Bonghan corpuscle (BHC): (a) at the moment of the microcapillary insertion into a cell membrane of a BHC. The potential decreases abruptly by about 38 mV from the reference potential of the bath. V_d is the potential drop. The potential increased slowly to the resting potential by 6.7 mV. V_e is the small increase, and T_e is the time of the increase (45.2 sec). The resting potential remained stable with fine background fluctuations, and the irregular activity of spontaneously evoked spikes in the resting potential arose for a duration (D_s) of about 16.6 seconds. (b) The spontaneous activity in the resting potential was examined more closely. The average amplitude (V_s) is 1.1 mV, and the average period (T_s) is 0.8 sec. (c) More magnified view of the spontaneous activity. A spike has an average half-width (F_s) of 0.27 seconds.

4.1. Measurement of the Resting Potential and Spontaneous Bioelectrical Potential of Primo Nodes and Vessels

Park recognized that the measurement of electrical signals was very important, because if Bonghan corpuscles and ducts are connected to each other and some liquid flows through the ducts, a driving force is necessary to deliver the liquid. According to this result, a resting potential and spontaneous action potential existed. They reported experimental values of −39.9 ±15.5 mV and 1.2 ±0.6 mV [37].

This result was highly significant as it was the first evidence that Bonghan corpuscles were composed of excitable cells and not types of fibrins and collagen fibers. In those days, almost every anatomical and histological expert insisted that Bonghan corpuscles and ducts are just collagen fibers and types of fibrins. So, the corpuscles and ducts are not only new structures but are nonfunctioning despite the fact that they may be new structures. However, his result showed that the spontaneous action potential was observed; thus, the corpuscle must have some special function.

Moreover, when the electrical signals were analyzed, the primary wave groups were 0.62–0.84 Hz, 0.36 Hz, 0.05 Hz, and 0.02 Hz (Figure 14). It is interesting to note that this is similar to the (geu), (neu), and (deu) wave forms reported by Kim in the 1960s [6, 24–27, 34].

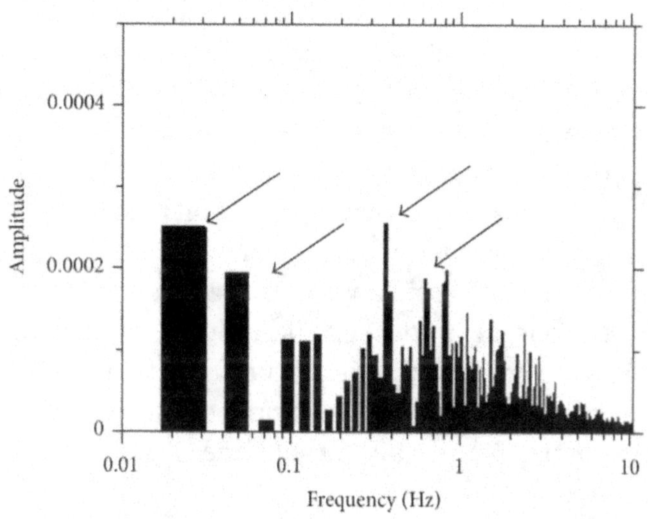

Figure 14
Fast Fourier transform (FFT) of the membrane potential. In this particular experiment, there were four values, 0.62–0.84 Hz, 0.36 Hz, 0.05 Hz, and 0.02 Hz, appearing above the broad background.

Choi developed a more precise experimental setup and experiment that measured the electrical potential from Bonghan ducts [44]. He was an oriental medical doctor and a physicist who thought that Bonghan corpuscles and ducts were not related to the Kyungrak system. In addition, he hypothesized that Bonghan ducts were types of fibrin and were similar to lymphatic vessels by conducting a comparison experiment.

However, he observed the resting potential (n = 17) and spontaneous action potential (n = 2) of Bonghan ducts, reporting a resting potential of -10.0 ± 4.7 mV from cells embedded in the surfaces of Bonghan ducts. He concluded the bioelectrical signals from Bonghan ducts and lymphatic vessels were different and that it would be pointless to discuss a comparison with fibrins. This was an important result which overturned his previous hypothesis, representing the first report of the resting potential and spontaneous action potential of Bonghan ducts (Figure 15) [44, 46]. There was some discussion about revising the nomenclature to expand the study of the Bonghan system around that time (Table 2).

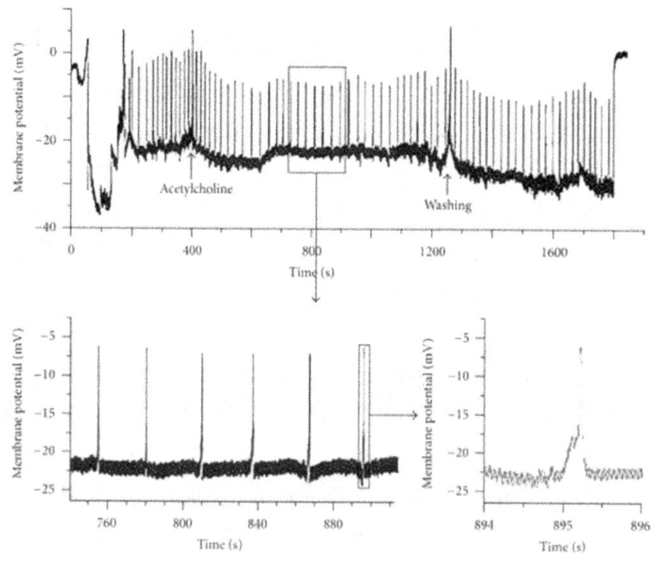

Figure 15

Spontaneous action potentials of the novel thread part. The resting potential was -22 mV; this is a quite unique value compared to that of other excitable cells. The bursting frequency decreased after applying acetylcholine and increased slightly after washing.

Table 2

Revised nomenclature for the Bonghan system.

Before	After
Bonghan system	Primo vascular system
Bonghan duct	Primo vessel
Bonghan corpuscle	Primo node
Bonghan liquor	Primo fluid
Bonghan sanal	Primo microcell

Open in a separate window

The intracellular recording method and the patch clamp method were used to measure the bioelectrical signals from Bonghan corpuscles and ducts by Choi [44]. He measured the electrical signals using a whole-cell slice-patch recording method for primo nodes and an intracellular recording method for primo vessels. His result reported a resting potential of –36.60 ±1.38 mV of the primo nodes but no spontaneous action potential. Small round cells are most abundant in primo nodes. On the basis of the current-voltage (I-V) relationships and kinetics of the outward currents, the cells of primo nodes could be grouped into four types. Among these, type I cells were the majority (69%) [43]. He reported that the resting potential of primo vessels was 21.0 ±2.2 mV and that there were two groups based on the resting potential (Type A (70%): –13.13 ±0.66 mV and Type B (30%): –38.64 ±2.96 mV). However, he reported that there were no properties of the spontaneous action potential of primo nodes and vessels, even if there were 2–4 cell groups (Figure 16) [43].

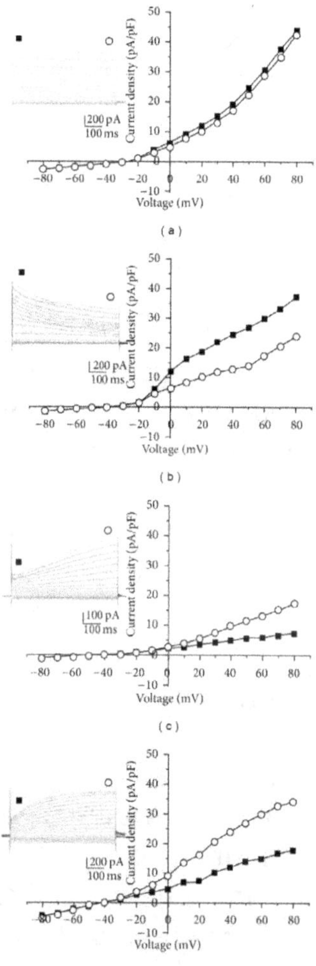

(a)

(b)

(c)

(d)

Figure 16

Four types of current-voltage (I.V) relationships recorded from cells in PN slices. I.V curves were obtained by depolarizing step pulses from −80 to 80 mV. (a) Type II.V relationships showing outward rectification. Note that the I.V relationships measured at 50 ms (solid squares) and 550 ms of the 600 ms current pulse (open circle) are identical. (b) Type III.V relationships showing outward rectification with the time-dependent activation of the outward current. (c) Type III I.V relationships showing outward rectification with a time-dependent and linearly activated outward current. Note the lower current density in this cell. (d) Type IV I.V relationships showing outward rectification with a time-dependent and hyperbolic increase in the outward current. The insets show the current traces for the I.V relationships in (a) and (d). The holding potential is −30 (a) and −40 mV (b and d). The largest outward tail current is seen in the current traces of the type IV cell. Scale bars for the insets are 10 μm.

The Korea Institute of Oriental Medicine began research on the primo vascular system in 2009. Lee et al. reported a method of distinguishing between torn mesentery and primo vessels [47]. Cho reported that there was the spontaneous action potential of primo vessels on internal organs using an extracellular recording method. The value of the potential was different from the action potential of a pacemaker of intestines. There were two types of cell groups reported as well [45].

Summarizing the research results pertaining to the resting potential and spontaneous action potential of primo nodes and vessels, resting potential and spontaneous action potential of cells from primo nodes and vessels and several cell type groups were discovered.

This conclusion was similar to the report of B. H. Kim, who found that there were distinct bioelectrical signals from the tissues of Bonghan corpuscles and ducts, also finding that modern electrophysiological technology could increase the confidence in results pertaining to the properties of bioelectrical signals from the primo vascular system.

4.2. Electrophysiological Study of the Primo Vascular System by Responding Drugs

Park was interested in the changing bioelectrical signals of Bonghan corpuscles by drug stimulation after measuring the resting potential and spontaneous action potential [37].

This was direct evidence that the Bonghan system may be a circulatory system such as the cardiac vascular system and the lymphatic system, because if there were excitable cells of the Bonghan system that responded to drugs, the system could contribute to the functions of the living body, like nerves and muscles. He attempted to find the response of bioelectrical signals from Bonghan corpuscles using acetylcholine, pilocarpine, atropine, and nifedipine. Acetylcholine is a major neurotransmitter in an autonomic nervous system. It stimulates both nicotinic and muscarinic receptors and is a common drug used to stimulate muscles. Pilocarpine is a nonselective muscarinic acetylcholine receptor agonist. Atropine is a cholinergic receptor antagonist and a competitive nonselective antagonist at central and peripheral muscarinic acetylcholine receptors. Consequently, as the electrical signals of Bonghan corpuscles respond to these drugs, Bonghan corpuscles have muscarinic receptors which are controlled by the autonomic nerve system. The Bonghan system may be an autonomic-nerve-controlled system.

Nifedipine is L-type Ca_{2+} channel blocker. The fundamental features of the spike generated in smooth muscles are related to the activation of the L-type Ca_{2+} channel. Ca_{2+} must be available for muscle contraction. Therefore, if there are Ca_{2+} ion channels in Bonghan corpuscles, it could be important evidence that Bonghan corpuscles have smooth muscle-like characteristics, such as contractibility and cell relaxation.

Park reported that the resting potential due to stimulation by acetylcholine was decreased to 50% and that the spike shape of the spontaneous action potentials completely changed [37]. Pilocarpine also changed the potential of Bonghan corpuscles similarly [48]. Although the corpuscles were stimulated by acetylcholine and pilocarpine, the resting potential of Bonghan corpuscles increased dramatically when stimulated by atropine (Figure 17) [37]. In the case of nifedipine stimulation, the resting potential also increased, though it decreased after stimulation with acetylcholine and pilocarpine. This was the first evidence of the existence of Ca_{2+} ion channels in the cell membranes of Bonghan corpuscles.

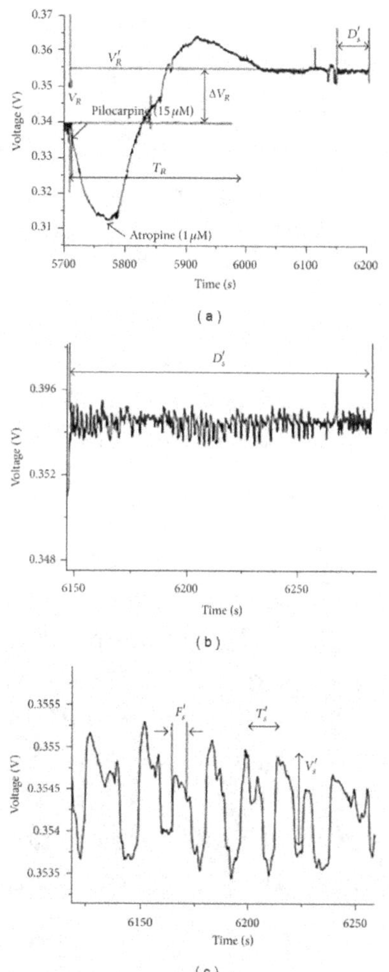

Figure 17

Effects of atropine on the resting potential and the spontaneous burst. (a) The resting potential dropped from V_R to V_R' and the decrease was ΔV_R. The resting potential slowly recovered its original value by ΔV_R. (b) The duration of the spontaneous burst ($D\ s'$). (c) The amplitude ($V\ s'$), period ($T\ s'$), and half width ($F\ s'$) of the spikes in the burst dramatically changed.

This result confirms that the Bonghan system may have the functions of contractibility and relaxation of the circulatory system [37]. Particularly, Park asserted that the electrical signals of smooth muscle-like cells from Bonghan corpuscles have similar properties to those of the vascular smooth muscle reported by Bkaily [49].

J. H. Choi studied the responses to drugs. He used tetraethylammonium (TEA). TEA is known to block the K+ channel in nerves and Ca2+ channels are also blocked [50, 51].

Tetraethylammonium (TEA) dose-dependently blocked both the outward and inward current (IC50, 4.3 mM at ±60 mV). Under current clamp conditions, TEA dose-dependently depolarized the membrane potential (18.5 mV at 30 mM) with an increase in the input resistance. These results demonstrate for the first time that a TEA-sensitive current with limited selectivity to K+ contributes to the resting membrane potential in type I cells [52].

In summary, in the previous results of drug stimulation experiments, primo nodes are shown to have muscarinic receptors, allowing the primo vascular system to be controlled by the autonomic nerve system. Moreover, the system has the possibility of contractibility and relaxation function due to the Ca_{2+} ion channels. Moreover, the cells of the primo vascular system may be excitable given the K_+ ion channels in the membranes of the cells. These results are in good agreement with the proteomics analyses of the primo vascular system [53].

Go to:

5. Discussion

The results of the bioelectrical signals and electrophysiology research are summarized in Tables

Tables3
3 and

and4.
4.

Table 3

A comparison of the electrophysiological characteristics between primo nodes, primo vessels, neurons, and muscle cells.

	RP (mV)	APD (mV)	Drug-responsive	Reference
Neuron	-70	1	Y	[19]

Muscle				
Skeletal	−80 to −90	2 to 5	Y	[20]
Cardiac	−85 to −95	200 to 400	Y	[21]
Smooth	−50 to −60	10 to 50	Y	[22]
Primo node				
Skin	·	0.1	Y	[25]
Surface of a small intestine	−39.9 to 15.5	1.2 to 0.6	Y	[37]
Surface of a small intestine	−36.6 to 1.38	·	Y	[43]
Primo vessel				
Skin	·	0.1	Y	[25]
Surface of a small intestine	−10 to 4.7	20 40	·	[44]
Surface of a small intestine	A: −13.1 to 0.7B: −38.6 to 3.0	·	Y	[43]
Surface of a small intestine	·	A: 10.0 to 8.4B: 13.7 to 8.7	·	[45]

Open in a separate window

RP: resting potential; TP: threshold potential; APD: action potential duration (bioelectrical activity).

Table 4

The summarization of the electrophysiological properties of the primo vascular system.

Target	Methodology	Cell Type	Result	Reference
Primo node	Intracellular recording	Vascular smooth muscle like	Excitable (Muscarinic receptor, Ca_{2+} ion channel)	[37]
	Patch clamp, Current-voltage relationship	Four types	Nonexcitable cell (K_+ ion channel for Type I)	[43]
	Extracelluar recording	Two types	Excitable cell (not smooth muscle like)	[45]
Primo duct	Intracellular recording	Smooth muscle Secreting cell Immune cell	Excitable Non-excitable	[44]

Open in a separate window

The bioelectrical study of primo nodes and vessels simply focused on the measurement of the resting potential and spontaneous action potential initially, as nobody knew whether the cells from the primo vascular system had intrinsic potentials or not. Therefore, it is important to confirm the properties of the action potential of cells related to the basic physiology functions.

While examining the papers related to the bioelectrical study of the primo vascular system, there were slight differences in the results of the resting potential, action potential, and the drugs responses depending on the study. The research is not sufficient for a complete understanding of the functions of the primo vascular system in the body precisely, but the primo vascular system clearly has excitable cells that respond to some stimuli.

The physiological functions of the primo vascular system should be confirmed by investigating the properties of each cell in the system and by measuring the resting potential and the action potential of each cell type. If each cell type of the primo vascular system could be determined, we will be able to understand the signal delivery methods and the conduction system.

Ultimately, the purpose of an electrical signal analysis of the primo vascular system is to investigate whether the internal substances of the primo nodes and primo vessels can be circulated. In addition, it is necessary to conduct additional experiments to answer the questions pertaining to the existence of an exclusive signal conduction system of the primo system circulation, like the nervous system, and to find evidence supporting the circulating function of the primo system based on actual mechanical activity. Research areas requested in the future may include the following:

1.   standardization of measured data by the standardization of techniques to measure the electrical signals of the primo vascular system;
2.   characterizing the cells composing the primo vascular system;
3.   investigating the electrical signal conduction and mechanical activity of the primo vascular system;
4.   uncovering the signal conduction mechanism through a connection between the primo vascular system and internal organs materially;
5.   investigating the control of the primo vascular system by external stimulation mechanisms such as medications and their interrelationships;
6.   looking into the circulation of internal substances inside the primo vascular system.

In addition, it is recommended to adopt useful technology to measure two-dimension spatial signal conduction methods such as optical electrophysiological techniques, which have greatly progressed recently, in addition to previous techniques of measuring one-dimension signals from a single point [54].

Though research on the electrical signals of the primo system started in the 1960s, the reliability of the study results was limited due to the limitations of the measuring technology and short descriptions of the methods and data. However, several studies of the electrophysiological characteristics of the primo vascular system have been performed since the 2000s, and it will be interesting to watch the development in the field of the electrophysiology of the primo vascular system in the future.

In conclusion, there are many differenct type cells composed of primo vascular system; one is the excitable cell type and the other is the nonexcitable cell type.

In case of the excitable cell, the vascular smooth muscle like cell type [37], the intestinal smooth muscle like cell type [45] and the immune cell type are reported

Advanced Glycation End Products: New Clinical and Molecular Perspectives

Juan Salazar,[1] Carla Navarro,[1] Ángel Ortega,[1] Manuel Nava,[1] Daniela Morillo,[2] Wheeler Torres,[1] Marlon Hernández,[3] Mayela Cabrera,[4] Lissé Angarita,[5] Rina Ortiz,[6] Maricarmen Chacín,[7] Luis D'Marco,[8,*] and Valmore Bermúdez[7,*]

José Carmelo Adsuar Sala, Academic Editor
Author information Article notes Copyright and License information PMC Disclaimer

Go to:

Abstract

Diabetes mellitus (DM) is considered one of the most massive epidemics of the twenty-first century due to its high mortality rates caused mainly due to its complications; therefore, the early identification of such complications becomes a race against time to establish a prompt diagnosis. The research of complications of DM over the years has allowed the development of numerous alternatives for diagnosis. Among these emerge the quantification of advanced glycation end products (AGEs) given their increased levels due to chronic hyperglycemia, while also being related to the induction of different stress-associated cellular responses and proinflammatory mechanisms involved in the progression of chronic complications of DM. Additionally, the investigation for more valuable and safe techniques has led to developing a newer, noninvasive, and effective tool, termed skin fluorescence (SAF). Hence, this study aimed to establish an update about the molecular mechanisms induced by AGEs during the evolution of chronic complications of DM and describe the newer measurement techniques available, highlighting SAF as a possible tool to measure the risk of developing DM chronic complications.

Keywords: advanced glycation end products, diabetes mellitus, chronic complications, skin fluorescence

Go to:

1. Introduction

Diabetes Mellitus (DM) is a metabolic disease characterized by chronic hyperglycemia due to absent or inadequate insulin secretion, combining with defective action on target tissues, depending on the type of diabetes [1]. DM has many categories; however, the main subtypes are type 1 diabetes mellitus (T1DM), type 2 diabetes mellitus (T2DM), and gestational diabetes mellitus [2]. Diabetes is currently considered one of the largest epidemics of the twenty-first century. In 2015, according to the International Diabetes Federation (IDF), 415 million people worldwide were estimated to have diabetes, and there were approximately 5 million deaths attributable to diabetes, which is estimated as a death every 6 s [3]. However, it is to emphasize that the leading cause of death is not diabetes per se but DM-derived complications that lead to systemic dysfunction [4].

As a result, the prompt identification of DM-associated complications has become significantly relevant. DM complications can be divided into two main types, acute and chronic complications. Acute complications involve hypoglycemia and hyperglycemic crises, which tend to onset abruptly [5], instead of the slow and steady progression of chronic complications over the years [6]. Regardless of the type of diabetes mellitus, the chronic complications are likewise divided into two categories depending on the vascular damage. Macrovascular complications include cardiovascular disease (CVD); meanwhile, microvascular complications include chronic kidney disease (CKD), neuropathy, and diabetic retinopathy [7].

Diverse studies have determined that advanced glycation end products (AGEs) are involved in the pathophysiological mechanisms of DM complications [8]. These derive from nonenzymatic reactions between carbohydrate residues and protein, lipids, or nucleic acids, along with oxidative processes [9]. The development mechanism of DM complications through AGEs is varied, since these can generate structural changes to different macromolecules, altering their function and leading to intracellular pathways that trigger inflammatory responses and endothelial damage [10]. Thus, measuring these changes works both as a diagnostic method of DM and as a biochemical marker of glycemic control, being the determination of hemoglobin A1c (HbA1c), the most known marker tested [11].

The quantification of AGEs can also serve to assess the risk of developing DM complications and measure their degree of progression [9]. Although multiple measurement techniques have been developed, the search for more accurate, selective, and safe procedures is still ongoing [11]. Luckily, skin fluorescence (SAF) has recently been described in several studies as a noninvasive method [12]. Here, we analyze the pathophysiological mechanisms induced by AGEs that trigger the progression of chronic complications of DM and describe the newer measurement techniques available, focusing on SAF, a possible tool to measure the risk of developing DM complications.

Go to:

2. Protein Glycation and Formation of Advanced Glycation End Products

Advanced glycation end products (AGEs) are an heterogeneous group of oxidative molecules with pathogenic capability [13]. The synthesis of these compounds begins with common metabolic pathways that occurred during the storage of food-derived products in the organism due to nonenzymatic reactions between reduced carbohydrates and free amino acids, peptides, lipids, or nucleic acids [14]. These reactions mentioned earlier are called Maillard reaction, glycation, or "nonenzymatic glycosylation" [15].

The generation of AGEs is completed through three stages [16], starting with the production of Schiff Bases [17], which emerge from the covalent bond established between the amino group of the free amino acid (generally composed by lysine and less frequently by arginine and cysteine residues), lipids, and nucleic acids with glucose [18,19]. This stage takes place in a time-lapse of hours following the postprandial glycemic increase, and it is characterized as a reversible reaction, since it can be re-established if the glycemic levels decrease [13].

Afterward, Schiff Bases submit to a molecular rearrangement, generating Amadori products, which are more stable compounds, although this stage is still reversible from carbohydrate oxidation [20]. The most recognized product is HbA1c, assembled through the junction of a valine residue of one of the β chain of this hemeprotein with plasma glucose [11]. Later, Amadori products accumulate in the organism; these go through reduction–oxidation reactions to eventually associate with secondary proteins through covalent bonds, altering their tertiary and quaternary structures and forming AGEs such as 3,4-*N*-carboxymethyl-lysine (CML), 3-deoxyglucosone (3DG), and Methylglyoxal (MG) [18]. AGEs have a brown-yellowish pigmentation, and some of them even have fluorescent properties, especially pyrrolidine, CML, imidazoline, and pentosidine [21]. Under physiological conditions, the glycation process occurs in weeks to years; nonetheless, in some pathological states such as hyperglycemia, oxidative stress, and temperature increase, the needed time can be reduced to hours [22] (Figure 1).

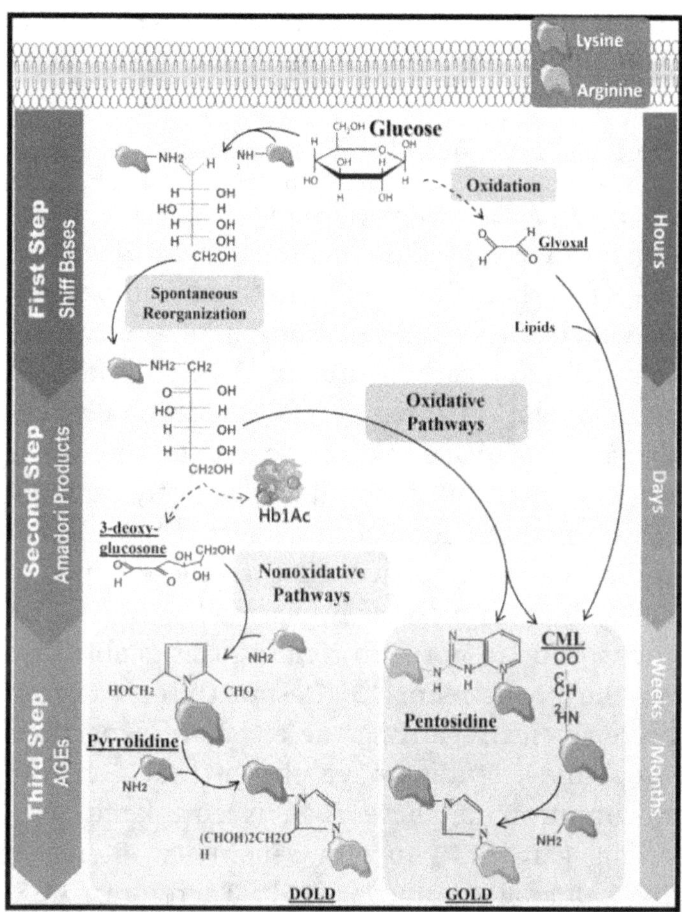

Figure 1

Maillard Reaction: production of AGEs. Production of AGEs initiates from a three-staged metabolic process denominated by a Maillard reaction, starting with the reversible formation of Schiff Bases, followed by a molecular rearrangement dnt that results in the generation of Amadori products and, finally, leading to the formation of AGEs due to a posterior binding to secondary proteins, establishing as nonreversible structures. This can occur due to oxidative processes such as the formation of pyrrolidine and, also, nonoxidative processes such as the formation of pentosidine and CML; however, other proteins can be added to these molecules, allowing the formation of products such as DOLD and GOLD. Additionally, there are alternative pathways to form AGEs; for instance, the oxidation of glucose and subsequent glyoxal formation can generate CML by the binding of glyoxal to lipids. Hb1Ac: glycated hemoglobin and CML: 3,4-*N*-carboxymethyl-lysine.

Comparatively, glucose has the slowest glycation rate of carbohydrate within these compounds, unlike fructose, glucose 6-phosphate, and threose (intracellular carbohydrates), which have a faster oxidation capacity [15]. Additionally, the formation of AGEs is also exogenous, since they can be found in food, like primarily animal-derived high-fat food such as beef [14]. Different studies have demonstrated that these types of food induce an increase in plasma levels of AGEs, since up to 10% of food rich in AGEs is absorbed into the bloodstream [13]. Despite the existence of discrepancies regarding the effects of exogenous compounds, studies have shown that a higher consumption of these food is correlated with weight gain [23], insulin sensitivity alteration [24], and albuminuria [25]. Therefore, AGE-rich diets, favoring oxidative stress and chronic inflammation states due to interactions with cellular compounds, are a substantial risk factor to the development of metabolic and cardiovascular complications [26].

Go to:

3. AGEs and Their Implication in Chronic

Complications of Diabetes Mellitus

Chronic complications of DM derive from structural and functional modifications of blood vessels due to hyperglycemia, affecting the heart, kidneys, and nervous system [27]. Among the mechanisms implied in developing these complications are the structural modifications induced by AGEs in vulnerable molecules such as proteins, lipids, and DNA, altering their stability and functions [28].

Activation of the receptor for advanced glycation end products (RAGE) represents the main mechanism involved between DM and AGEs [8]. RAGE is a cell surface receptor composed of three extracellular domains, a transmembrane domain, and a cytoplasmic tail [8], which belongs to the immunoglobulin superfamily [29], since its expression derives from the major histocompatibility complex class III (MHC-III) [30]. Thus, RAGE expression predominates in specific cells such as monocytes, macrophages, proximal tubular cells, podocytes, and mesangial cells [29].

As a result of the AGE–RAGE interaction, the cytoplasmic domain of RAGE leads to different signaling pathways. In particular, it can activate the p21 protein [31], triggering other signaling compounds to eventually stimulate kinases such as the extracellular signal-regulated kinase (ERK), c-Jun *N*-terminal kinase (JNK), and mitogen-activated protein kinase (MAP) [29], along with Janus kinase 1 and 2/Signal transducer and activators of transcription (JAK/STAT1) [32]. Finally, the consequences of these signal transduction pathways consist of the activation of transcription factors such as nuclear factor kappa B (NF-kB) [33] and the interferon-sensitive response element (ISRE) [34], which lead to the synthesis of proinflammatory cytokines as tumor necrosis factor-alpha (TNF-α) [34] and interleukins (IL) 1, 6, and 17 [35,36], as well as vascular cell adhesion molecule-1 (VCAM-1) [29].

Additionally, NADH oxidase's activation directly and indirectly generates reactive oxygen species (ROS) due to RAGE stimulation [37]. Furthermore, RAGE can be activated by other types of ligands aside from AGEs, including S 100 or Calgranulin, Mac-1, High-mobility group box 1 (HMBG1), and β-amyloids, predominantly when their levels increase during inflammatory reactions (Figure 2) [31]. The discovery of RAGE's multiligand nature explains its elevated and persistent activity in diabetes complications [36,37].

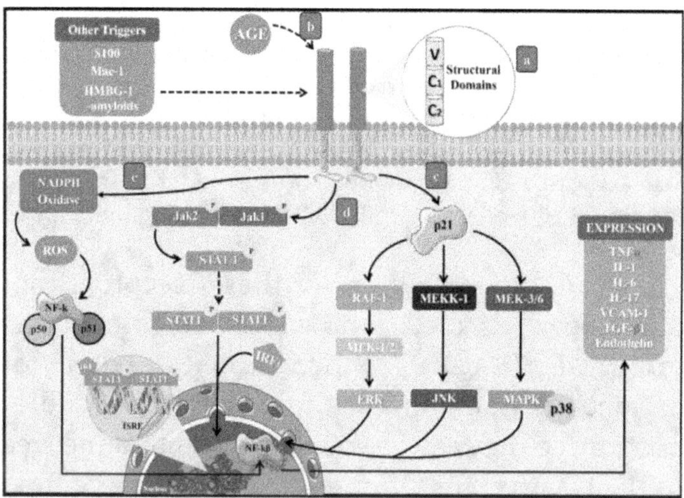

Figure 2

Signaling pathways induced by the activation of the receptor of AGEs. (**a**) RAGE is a cell surface receptor composed of three extracellular domains, a transmembrane domain, and a short cytoplasmic tail. (**b**) AGEs bind to RAGE's extracellular portion and induce activation of the cytoplasmic domain, leading to different signaling pathways, which will finally result in the stimulation of transcription factors such as NF-KB and ISRE. Three pathways that can lead to such a response: (**c**) activation of the protein p21, which induces RAF-1, MEKK-1, and MEK 3/6 proteins that activate the factors ERK, JNK, and MAPK, which translocate to the cell nucleus. (**d**) Activation of the JAK2/STAT1 pathway, where STAT1 dimerizes and binds to the IRF1 sequence to translocate to the cell nucleus, binding to the ISRE segment and inducing transcription of proinflammatory cytokines. (**e**) Activation of the NADPH oxidase that leads to the stimulation of NF-KB. These processes can be activated by other molecules such as S100, Mac-1, HMBG-1, and β-amyloids. NF-kB: nuclear factor kappa light chain enhancer of activated B cells, ISRE: interferon-sensitive response element, TNFα: tumor necrosis factor-alpha, IL: interleukins, VCAM-1: adherence and growth factors as the vascular cell adhesion molecule-1, TGF-β1: transforming growth factor β, RAF-1: proto-oncogene serine/threonine kinase, MEKK-1: mitogen-activated protein kinase kinase kinase 1, MEK 3/6: mitogen-activated protein kinase kinase, ERK: extracellular signal-regulated kinase, JNK: c-Jun N-terminal kinase, MAPK: mitogen-activated protein kinase, JAK: Janus kinase, STAT: signal transducer and activators of transcription, IRF1: interferon regulatory factor-1, S 100: calgranulin, and HMBG1: high-mobility group box 1.

There are different types of these receptors that have been studied, known as soluble forms of RAGE (RAGEs), which are composed of extracellular domains without their intracellular portion, so they can be transported and found free in the plasma [38]. Of note, two types of receptors have been identified, cleaved RAGE(cRAGE) and endogenous secretory RAGE (esRAGE) or RAGE_V1, depending on how they were created [39]. cRAGE is formed from the action of matrix metalloproteases (MMP) and α-disintegrin metalloprotease (ADAM)-10; these enzymes cleave from the cell surface to RAGE, thus losing its transmembrane and cytosolic portions, but it conserves the V1-C1-C2 domains of RAGE. On the other hand, esRAGE is generated by the alternative splicing of the RNAm RAGE gene, changing its structure by adding a 16-amino acid extension at the c-terminal end [40].

Although the distribution and function of these receptors are not yet clear, there are multiple hypotheses about their role in the pathophysiology of inflammatory and metabolic diseases, such as DM. Among the most managed actions, their role as "decoys" for AGEs is evaluated, generating a downregulation effect in inflammation and preventing cell damage due to the sequestration of RAGE ligands that leads to the pathways not activated being intracellularly related to these receptors not only by AGEs but other ligands such as HMB1 or S100, postulating a possible regulatory action on the AGEs–RAGE axis [40]. In addition, studies have established an inversely proportional relationship between the levels of sRAGE and the markers of metabolic syndrome and atherosclerosis in patients with DM, used as a biomarker in inflammatory processes and complications associated with this disease [41].

3.1. Molecular Mechanisms of AGEs in Microvascular Complications of DM

The presence of diabetic retinopathy, neuropathy, or (micro) albuminuria defines the existence of microvascular complications of DM [42]; despite affecting different organs, these complications mutually relate to each other [43]. Diverse studies have associated AGEs with the progression of those complications, mainly given the direct action of these products on tissues or via stimulation of the AGE–RAGE axis and the subsequent inflammatory response [44,45,46].

Diabetic kidney disease (DKD) is characterized by renal hypertrophy, proteinuria, decreased glomerular filtration rate, and renal fibrosis [47], ultimately progressing to chronic kidney disease (CDK) [48]. Induction of the AGE–RAGE pathways deriving from the accumulation of these products in renal tissue leads to inflammatory activity [49]. Thus, triggering the migration of macrophages that agglomerate in the renal glomerulus's mesangium and establishing an inflammatory microenvironment led by IL-6 synthesis with the consequent expansion of this layer eventually causes the compression of capillaries and reduction of the body surface area of renal filtration [50]. Additionally, increased expression of transforming growth factor β (TGF-β) has been correlated with fibrogenesis activation, collagen synthesis stimulation, and renal tubular cell apoptosis, therefore explaining both glomerular sclerosis and dysfunction [51].

Other mechanisms induced by the AGE–RAGE pathway arise specifically through CML, which constitutes a higher AGE accumulation in vivo [52], the renal epithelium being continuously exposed to these changes [53]. It has been recently determined that AGEs generate lipid accumulation in this tissue deriving from altered cholesterol metabolism, since AGEs activate the sterol-regulatory element-binding protein 2 (SREBP-2) and, correspondingly, the expression of 3-hydroxy-3-methylglutaryl-coenzyme A reductase (HMG-CoA reductase) increases, concluding in an increased cholesterol synthesis. Additionally, this molecule's access to cells benefits from the stimulation of low-density lipoprotein (LDLc) activity in conjunction with the decrease of the ATP-binding cassette transporter A1 (ABCA1), which results in tissue dysfunction [44] (Figure 3).

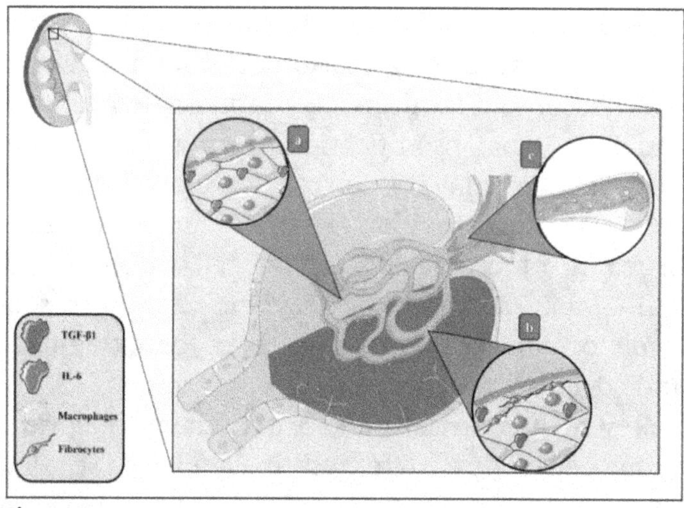

Figure 3

AGEs in diabetic kidney disease. Activation of the AGE–RAGE axis derived from the accumulation of AGEs in renal tissue induces tissue dysfunction through diverse mechanisms: (a) macrophage migration, which agglomerates in the renal glomerulus's mesangium, establishing an inflammatory microenvironment led by IL-6 synthesis and, eventually, causing the expansion of this layer, compression of the capillary, and reduction of the body surface area of filtration. (b) Increased expression of transforming growth factor β

(TGF-β), which stimulates fibrogenesis, collagen synthesis, and renal tubular cell apoptosis, leading to glomerular sclerosis. (c) Lipids storage from altered cholesterol metabolism as a result of the activation of sterol-regulatory element-binding protein 2 (SREBP-2), increasing the expression of 3-hydroxy-3-methylglutaryl-coenzyme A reductase (HMG-CoA reductase) and, finally, concluding in increased cholesterol synthesis.

Diabetic neuropathy is defined by the progressive loss of axons within peripheral nerves, clinically manifested by severe pain and sensory impairment [54]. The accumulation of AGEs in the endoneurium, Schwann cells, extracellular matrix, and capillary within these nervous structures cause the glycation of proteins such as fibronectin and laminin [55], inducing structural and functional modifications that decrease the regenerative capacity related to axonal atrophy [56]. Likewise, oxidative stress and, thereby, neuronal cytotoxicity are induced through the AGE–RAGE pathway [57], given the increased levels of superoxide and hydrogen peroxide [58] and decreased intracellular glutathione (GSH) [46], which is an essential antioxidant tripeptide composed of glutamate, cysteine, and glycine [59].

The loss of peripheral sensation and the increase of mechanical pressure in the feet are the primary cause of diabetic foot [60]. Secondly, the oxidative stress, proinflammatory cytokines presence, and glycation of proteins such as collagen lead to the hardening of epithelial cells 'basement membranes, concluding in skin tissue frailty and impaired wound healing [61].

On the other hand, diabetic retinopathy (DR) constitutes a degenerative vascular process that progresses through different stages [62]. First, a blood flow imbalance emerges, in addition to an increased vascular permeability and capillary basement membrane hardening, advancing to the formation of microaneurysms and establishing a microvascular injury that produces ischemia due to decreased retinal blood flow, thus representing a significant cause of blindness [63,64]. The development of these pathological changes results from pericyte apoptosis induced by the AGE–RAGE pathway. Likewise, increased oxidative stress produced by NF-kB expression produces free radicals such as peroxynitrite inside the subretinal membrane and microvasculature, damaging the DNA [65].

Moreover, the regulatory function of Müller cells inside the retina [66] becomes affected in DM by exposure to hyperglycemia [67], and the inflammatory process, alongside its effects on the microvasculature, is also a consequence of activation of the AGE–RAGE pathway [45]. Furthermore, this pathway increases the expression of cytokines and proangiogenic factors such as the vascular endothelial growth factor (VEGF) [68], basic fibroblast growth factor (bFGF) [69], and TGF-β [70], leading to the distinguished neovascularization of DR and significantly exacerbated by the high accumulation capacity of AGEs in the vitreous humor [69].

3.2. AGEs and the Macrovascular Alterations in DM

Cardiovascular complications of DM arise as a consequence of the damage to large-diameter vascular structures. They are mostly the leading cause of death among diabetic patients, representing 50% of the deaths related to this disease [27]. Diabetic cardiomyopathy is characterized by ventricular dysfunction originating from myocyte hypertrophy [71,72] and myocardial fibrosis [73]. The AGE–RAGE axis has been admitted as one of the contributing factors to this incompletely elucidated chronic complication (**Figure 4**) [29].

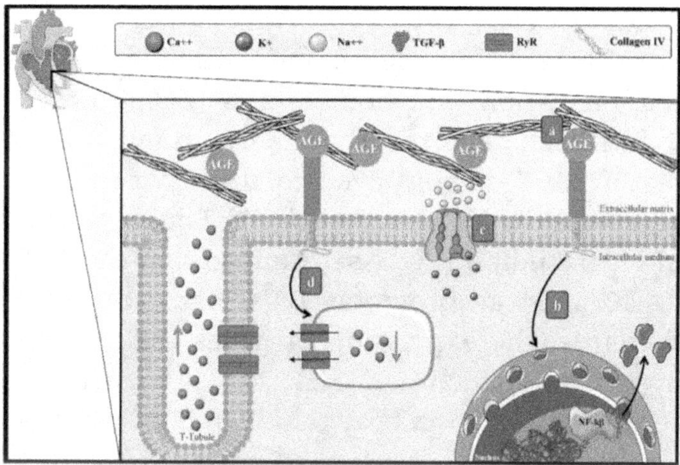

Figure 4

AGEs in diabetic cardiomyopathy. The effect of the AGEs in diabetic cardiomyopathy arises through diverse mechanisms: (**a**) accumulation in the extracellular matrix of cardiac tissue due to the interaction with structural proteins, inducing reticulation between collagen fibers and laminin and decreasing the elastic properties of the cardiac tissue. (**b**) Activation of the AGE–RAGE pathway by the induction of TGF-β and other proinflammatory cytokines that allow the proliferation of fibroblasts conducive to myocardial hypertrophy. (**c**) Activation of the AGE–RAGE pathway and ionic imbalance due to inhibition of the SIRT1/NAD+ pathway, disturbing the function of the Na++/K+ ATPase. (**d**) Overstimulation of the RyR, generating irregular modifications of the Ca++ levels, favoring its exit and causing an alteration of the cardiac cycle that advances to diastolic dysfunction. Ca++: calcium, K+: potassium, Na++: sodium, TGF-β1: transforming growth factor β, and RyR: ryanodine receptors.

This process may cause the deterioration of cardiac functions by myocyte hypertrophy [74]. Lately, it has been established that this cardiac remodeling process occurs through the connection within the AGE–RAGE pathway and dendritic cells (DC) [75], which are antigen-presenting cells with essential functions in T-cell regulation and homeostasis [76]. However, it has been reported that the accumulation of matured DC during myocardial infarction could aggravate the tissue remodel [77]. Equally, during in vitro studies, it was determined that the AGE–RAGE pathway promotes DC's maturation and, therefore, the expression of genes that develop hypertrophy, such as *MYH7*, which encodes the cardiac beta-myosin heavy chain (β-MHC) [75,78].

The increment in fibroblast numbers after the increase of AGEs in the extracellular matrix [74] promotes interactions with structural proteins, inducing reticulation between collagen fibers and laminin, deriving in a loss of the cardiac tissue's elastic properties, rigidity, and increased cardiac volume, conductive to diastolic dysfunction [79,80]. The AGE–RAGE pathway intervenes in fibroblast proliferation by stimulating proinflammatory genes and TGF-β, amplifying the adverse effect on the cardiac elastic properties [81].

Separately, the accumulation of AGEs in cardiac tissue is also related to the inhibition of the sirtuin-1 protein (SIRT1) expression. SIRT1, a member of the class III deacetylase family, is an antioxidant protein capable of delaying fibrosis and apoptosis of cardiac cells through its activation by NAD+ [82]. Besides, the adenosine monophosphate-activated protein kinase (AMPK) keeps a cellular energetic balance and enhances the NAD+ levels and can also regulate SIRT1 functions [83]. In conclusion, it has been established that Na++/K+ ATPase alterations are due to dysregulation of the SIRT1/AMPK pathway, modifying cellular ionic homeostasis [84].

Moreover, the Ca2+ levels decrease due to the increased activity of the ryanodine receptors induced by AGE–RAGE [85]. These receptors manage to equilibrate the ion levels during diastole and systole [86]; however, their hyperactivity allows a Ca2+ leak from the sarcoplasmic reticulum during diastole, diminishing the Ca2+ levels during systole and, thus, disturbing the cardiac cycle [87], driving to cardiac dysfunction [85].

Go to:

4. Progression of Measurement Techniques of AGEs in Patients with DM

Numerous studies have determined the essential role of the plasma levels of AGEs in developing chronic DM complications [29,88,89,90], being described as even better markers than the HbA1c measurements [91]. Experimentally, it has been observed that preventing these products' accumulation reduces the development and progression of DM-associated complications. As a result, different measurement techniques have been developed to quantify AGEs, including biochemical and immunohistochemical methods capable of measuring products such as pentosidine and CML [92].

The plasma levels of AGEs come from the balance between the synthesis of circulating proteins, accumulation in different tissues [93], absorption from food [14], and renal clearance [94]. For this reason, urine and blood samples allow quantifying their levels that are relevant in DN, especially during the end stage of the disease [95]. The most used measurement technique is the enzyme-linked immunosorbent assay (ELISA), which relies on AGE-recognizing antibodies (Ac), mediated through their bindings and their posterior identification using fluorescence techniques [96]. In this regard, Münch et al. initially described ELISA and validated two procedures: the use of direct monoclonal Ac, which can specifically recognize imidazoline, a product derived from the union of arginine with 3-deoxyglucosone. Secondly, since that technique's development, different measurement methods using prepared Ac that recognize the epitopes of various AGEs have been designed, including CML [8,96,97].

Nevertheless, applying these types of measurements has been disputed due to both difficulties in reproducing and determining AGE epitopes that can interact with the specific Ac [98]. Thus, the interest in quantifying diabetic patients' AGEs through their fluorescent properties has increased [21]. Recently, high-performance liquid chromatography (HPLC) analyzes the components of a mixture made by the interaction between the used substances and chromatography columns [99] and can determine the levels of AGEs according to the intensity of their fluorescence. HPLC also allows a faster analysis of protein-bound AGEs such as pentosidine [21] while establishing their influence on the tissues 'biologic characteristics [21].

The use of mass spectrometry (MS) has also been incorporated; this tool allows to identify, characterize, and quantify chemical compounds depending on fragmentation patterns [100]. In this regard, gas chromatography-mass spectrometry (GC-MS) [101] is used as a specific method to quantify oxidative stress markers [102], detecting the activity of products such as CML in heart failure and increasing its association with mortality [101]. Thus, demonstrating the impact of oxidative stress upon these diseases may improve the antioxidant therapy efficacy [103,104]. Likewise, liquid chromatography-MS (LC-MS) [105] has also been developed, granting a more straightforward way to use MS while reducing the limitations presented by GC-MS [100]. This technique allows the determination of plasma levels of AGEs according to DM evolution, exhibiting high levels since the early stages [106], besides their protein-damaging activity in conjunction with other oxidative processes [107], estimating their measure to prevent the development of chronic complications of DM [106].

Despite these techniques 'exceptional results, there are still concerns regarding their cost, complexity, and fluctuations among their results [108]. There is the requirement of newer techniques with more uncomplicated applications and higher reliability [108].

Go to:

5. Measurement of Skin Fluorescence

It has been demonstrated that AGEs heavily conglomerate within tissue structures, specifically inside skin collagen [91]. In this context, a notable difference between tissue and plasma measurement results has been observed [109], the skin collagen being the highest concentration location, thus correlating with the presence and severity of DM's chronic complications [110]. Hence, the measurement of tissue's AGEs has become more meaningful, including assessing the cornea, lens [111], or even a skin biopsy [112]. Moreover, there have been techniques designed concerning skin fluorescence and the presence of

AGEs in dermis structures [108].

In this regard, Meerwaldt et al. developed an instrument capable of measuring skin fluorescence (SAF) in a noninvasive modality and comparing the autofluorescence reader (AFR) results with the results obtained through skin biopsies; they determined its effectivity, validating the application of SAF as a method to quantify AGEs in DM [108].

The SAF principle relies on the relation between skin fluorescence and the presence of AGEs (Figure 5) [108], explaining its application as a marker to assess the chronic complications of DM [113,114,115,116,117]. Considering that skin collagen's half-life is about 10–15 years [118], the AGEs bound to skin collagen throughout such a time are a medium to represent the maintained glycemia during long periods [113]. Furthermore, a retrospective study determined that a positive correlation exists between the SAF and HbA1c values measured every three months in patients with DM1, demonstrating a correlation between SAF and long-term glycemic control [119].

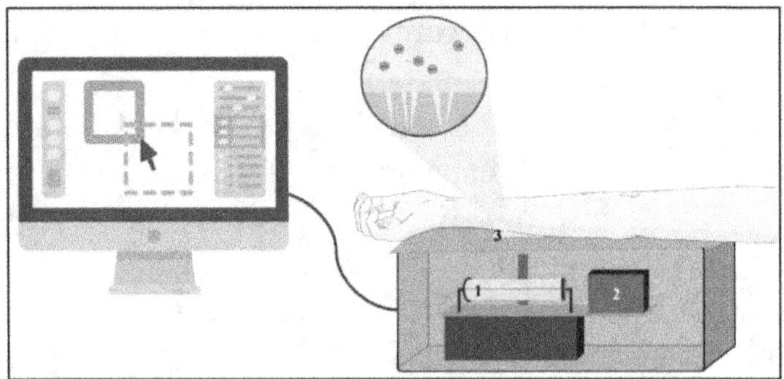

Figure 5

From the surface: the interior of the Skin Autofluorescence Reader. The Skin Autofluorescence Reader consists of a tube that illuminates UV radiation with an intensity of 300–420 nm upon approximately 1 cm2 of skin, which must not have scars or other abnormalities. The test must be performed in a semi-dark environment to avoid light interference. Said stimulus excites AGEs, which are bound to skin proteins and have autofluorescent properties within that range. These emit their fluorescence from light waves within a range of 420–600 nm and can be detected by a spectrometer. The autofluorescence of the stimulated AGEs is measured by the proportion between the intensity of the emitted light (420–600 nm) and the excitation light (300–420 nm) multiplied by 100, aiming to compensate for the effect of the skin pigmentation in the capacity of light absorption on the autofluorescence. The obtained results are expressed in arbitrary units (AU) and are shown immediately in a computed connected to the measurer, with a reference established from the results considering the patient's age. (1) Source of UV light, (2) spectrometer, and (3) illumination window.

While the implementation of SAF to measure the concentration of AGEs in tissue increased, some limitations arose. Among them, skin pigmentation [120], since the measurements in dark skin patients resulted in lower values than patients of Caucasian origin, attributed to the decreased absorption of excitatory or emitted lights from the skin components [121]. For instance, melanin can decrease UV radiation penetration through the epidermis [122], impairing the recognition of fluorescence emitted by AGEs in skin proteins [108].

Based on these findings, Kooetsier et al. validated an algorithm that allows the evaluation of SAF in individuals of different skin colors; contrastingly, this adjustment has solely been applied in healthy individuals [121,123]; in consequence, more research regarding its application on sick patients, mainly with DM, and its complications is required.

Go to:

6. Therapeutic Strategies: Halting the AGE–RAGE Axis

The discovery of the pleiotropic effects of AGEs in the establishment and progression of micro- and macrovascular complications of DM [29] has driven the search for prompt intervention strategies on the advanced glycation pathway that can diminish the damage upon target organs and improve the quality of life of affected patients [124]. Thus, lifestyle modifications and better glycemic control are still the key to prevent the first steps of the AGE process [125]. Indeed, it has been proven an the AGE-rich diet consumption restriction [23,24] added to smoking cessation [126,127] are measurements capable of significantly decreasing the serum levels of CML and MG, with beneficial effects on the skin fluorescence values, respectively. Similarly, it has been reported that an increase of the energy requirements induced by regular physical activity could improve glycemic control and reduce the availability of reactive precursors for glycation reactions, decreasing the accumulation of AGEs in diabetic patients [128].

Nevertheless, over the last few decades, there has been an exhaustive study of pharmacologic agents capable of interfering with the diverse glycation process stages, demonstrating promising results in numerous models in vitro and in vivo [129]. These drugs 'mechanisms of action rely principally on inhibiting the absorption of exogenous AGEs, preventing their endogenous formation and inducing the rupture of preformed AGEs or antagonizing their union with their receptor (Table 1) [130,131,132,133,134,135,136].

Table 1

Recent clinical evidence of therapeutic interventions in advanced glycation products and their complications.

Mechanism of Action	Drug	Methodology	Results	Author [REF]
Inhibition of the endogenous formation	Benfotiamine and Pyridoxamine	Randomized, double-blinded controlled	Significant decrease in serum levels and	Garg S et al. (2013) [130]

of AGEs		by placebo trial, which included 30 patients with primary osteoarthritis divided randomly between two groups to receive tablets of inhibitors of AGEs (benfotiamine (50 mg) + PM (50 mg) + methylcobalamin (500 mg)) or placebo tablets, three times a day.	fluorescence of AGEs. Decreased pain and inflammation. Increase in daily activity and mobility in patients with osteoarthritis.	
	Pioglitazone and Metformin	Randomized, open parallel-groups trial, performed in patients recently diagnosticated with DM2, who were given 30 mg/day of pioglitazone (n = 30), 1000 mg/day of metformin (n = 50) or not any drugs (n = 49).	In both treated groups with either pioglitazone or metformin was observed a statistically significant decrease in levels of AOPP and AGEs, besides causing an increase in FRAP (a marker of plasma antioxidant capacity).	Mirmiranpour H et al. (2013) [131]

Enalapril and Lercanidipine	Randomized, double-blinded trial, which included 359 ambulatory patients <65 years of age, first-diagnosed with essential hypertension and without treatment, divided between three groups, who were randomly given: enalapril 20 mg/day (n = 126), lercanidipine 10 mg/day (n = 115), or enalapril + lercanidipine 20/10 mg/day (118), in order to assess their effects in markers of cardiovascular risk.	All treatments showed a significant increase in levels of sRAGE, which was higher in patients treated with enalapril + lercanidipine. Significant reduction of levels of TNF-α and US-CRP in patients treated with enalapril + lercanidipine	Derosa G et al. (2014) [132]
Benfotiamine	Randomized, double-blinded, controlled trial, which included 41 patients	Patients treated with benfotiamine had a statistically significant decrease in	Contreras C et al. (2017) [133]

		with DM2 without complicatio ns, who were randomly given 900 mg/day of benfotiamin e or 900 mg/ day of a placebo, to assess their effect on levels of AGEs and sRAGE.	levels of carboxymeth yl-lysine. There were no statistically significant differences in levels of sRAGE.	
Breakage and Reversal of preformed AGEs	Alagebrium (ALT-711)	Randomized , double-blinded, controlled by placebo prospective study, performed in 57 healthy subjects over 60 years of age, which were randomly divided between 4 groups: sedentary + placebo, sedentary + alagebrium (200 mg/ day), exercise + placebo, and exercise + alagebrium in order to assess their	Alagebrium led to a moderate improvemen t in rigidity of the left ventricle, which was more prominent when it was combined with physical activity.	Fujimoto N et al. (2013) [134]

		effect in hemodynam ics, function, and structure of the left ventricle.		
	Alagebrium	Randomized , controlled by placebo trial, which included 47 older subjects previously sedentary, who were divided between 4 types of intervention s: Exercise + Alagebrium (200 mg/ day), Exercise + Placebo, Alagebrium (200 mg/ day), and Exercise aiming to examine their effect over endothelial function, arterial stiffness, and cardiovascul ar risk.	There were no improvemen ts in endothelial function or arterial stiffness in any of the four groups.	Oudegeest -Sander M et al. (2013) [135]
Inhibition of the absorption of exogenous	Sevelamer carbonate	Randomized , open, single- blinded trial,	Patients treated with sevelamer carbonate	Yubero- Serrano et al. (2015) [136]

AGEs		which included 117 patients with T2DM and diabetic nephropathy in stages 2 to 4, who were given sevelamer carbonate (1600 mg) or calcium carbonate (1200 mg), three times a day, to measure their effects in the AGE–RAGE axis and onto oxidative stress.	showed a significant reduction of both circulating and intracellular AGEs (carboxymethyl-lysine and methylglyoxal). It was also observed a significant increase in antioxidant defenses and reduction of pro-oxidant molecules.

Open in a separate window

AGEs, advanced glycation end products; AOPP, advanced oxidation protein products; T2DM, Type 2 diabetes mellitus; FRAP, Ferritin reducing ability of plasma; HbA1C, glycated hemoglobin; RAGE, receptor for advanced glycation end products; sRAGE, soluble RAGE; TNF-α, tumor necrosis factor-α; US-CRP, ultra-sensitive C-Reactive Protein; and sVCAM, soluble vascular cell adhesion molecule-1.

6.1. Inhibition of the Absorption of Exogenous AGEs

Studying inhibitory compounds of the absorption of AGEs acquires relevance by considering the limitations surrounding the implementation of strict diet modifications to decrease these proinflammatory compounds 'exogenous sources. One particular agent researched to accomplish this issue is AST-120 (Kremezin) [137], an oral adsorbent drug composed of porous spherical carbonic particles mainly indicated for treating patients with CKD to attenuate its progression by removing uremic toxins inside the bowels [138]. AST-120 has been described as capable of binding to food's CML in the bowels, impairing its absorption. As a result, a significant reduction of the serum levels of AGEs has been reported, aside from decreasing the ARNm of RAGE, the monocyte chemoattractant protein-1 (MCP-1), and the vascular cell adhesion molecule-1 (VCAM-1) in endothelial cells, diminishing the inflammatory response induced by these molecules [139]. On the other hand, sevelamer carbonate, a nonabsorbable oral drug used primarily as a phosphate binding agent to prevent hyperphosphatemia in patients with CKD [140], has proven to prevent the absorption of diet AGEs, in addition to decreasing the serum and cellular levels of AGEs and other inflammation markers [141].

6.2. Inhibition of the Endogenous Formation of AGEs

To date, the most widely studied drugs are precisely those destined to impede endogenous AGE formation. The first drug developed to achieve this purpose was aminoguanidine (AG) [142], a compound of hydralazine that, in virtue of its guanidine group, is capable of trapping α-dicarbonyl compounds such as MG and 3DG produced during the glycation early stage and, therefore, can prevent their subsequent reaction with amino groups of proteins [143,144]. The outcome described above has been correlated to a significant attenuation of chronic complications of diabetes [145], such as atherosclerosis, DN, retinopathy, and neuropathy, in numerous experimental studies [146,147]. Accordingly, studies have focused on elucidating the inhibitory properties of the AGE formation of bioactive compounds derived from herbs and spices [148], along with multiple drugs used in clinical practice —specifically, for instance, metformin [149], the vitamin B complex, and even antihypertensive drugs such as the angiotensin-converting enzyme inhibitors (ACEI) and angiotensin II receptor blockers (ARBs) [150].

Concerning phytochemicals, through the inhibition of AGE precursors, experimental studies have determined an antiglycation effect of polyphenols and other bioactive compounds extracted from plant species such as *Cinnamomum verum J.* (Ceylon-Cinnamon), *Syzygium aromaticum L.* (Cloves), *Pimpinella anisum L.* (Anise), *Pimenta dioica L.* (Allspice), *Rumex japonicus*, *Ilex paraguarieusis*, *Piper auritum*, and *Origanum majorana* [151,152,153,154]. Although the mechanisms behind the antiglycation effect are not precisely known [155], it has been reported that compounds such as resveratrol, oxyresveratrol, and piceatannol can inhibit the production of AGEs through the elimination of reactive carbonyl species [156].

Metformin, a biguanide extensively used as an antihyperglycemic drug for treating patients with DM2 [157], has recently been linked to important antioxidant and anti-inflammatory properties [158,159]. Using metformin as an inhibitor of AGEs is justified due to its structural similarity to AG, and it has also been proven capable of reacting with α-dicarbonyl compounds [160], preventing the posterior production of AGEs [161].

Contrarily, vitamins such as pyridoxamine (PM), thiamine pyrophosphate, and its lipophilic derivative benfotiamine have been demonstrated to intervene during the late stage of the glycation process, blocking the transformation of Amadori products into AGEs [162,163]; however, their actions are carried out throughout different levels. PM traps reactive oxygen species, leading to the blockage of the oxidative degradation of Amadori intermediaries while promoting the elimination of toxic carbonyl products originating from glucose and lipid degradation [164,165,166]. Differently, thiamine pyrophosphate and benfotiamine increase the transketolase activity, an enzyme that reduces the accumulation of glycolytic metabolites like glyceraldehyde-3-phosphate and fructose-6-phosphate by stimulating the pentose phosphate pathway, both involved in the formation of intracellular AGEs [163].

Another form to impede the formation of AGEs depends on the chelation of transition metals [167] such as Mg_{2+}, Cu_{2+}, and Zn_{2+}, since, during hyperglycemic conditions, these function as catalysts of oxidation reactions, thus favoring the formation of AGEs [168]. Regarding this, it has been found that the inhibitory actions on the formation of AGEs shown by some antihypertensive agents such as losartan and valsartan [169,170] can be attributed to their antioxidant and metal-chelating properties, which have also been associated with the decreased plasma levels of AGEs in various experimental studies [171].

6.3. Breakage and Reversal of Preformed AGEs

Other sorts of compounds have obtained relevance throughout the search for inhibitors of the glycation pathway. These are the *N*-phenacylthiazolium bromide (PTB) [172] with its derivative ALT-711 or alagebrium (dimethyl-3-*N*-phenacylthiazolium chloride) [173], given their ability to cleave AGE-AGE crosslinks that maintain AGEs attached to tissue proteins like collagen and elastin [174]. Thoroughly, their precise mechanisms of action rely on their reactions to carbonyl groups located in the crosslinks between AGEs, subsequently promoting the spontaneous cleavage of carbon–carbon bonds at physiologic pH [175]. Likewise, an experimental study demonstrated the efficacy of MnmC, an enzyme involved in bacterial tRNA modification, capable of performing a catalytic reversion of the AGEs carboxyethyl-lysine (CEL) and carboxymethyl-lysine (CML) to lysine's native structure [176]. The application of these drugs, mainly alagebrium, in diverse animal models has proven to be helpful in arterial stiffness reduction, blood vessel fibrosis [173,177], the development of atherosclerosis [178], cardiovascular disease [179], hypertension [180], and kidney injury [181].

6.4. Antagonism towards RAGE-Binding

Finally, agents capable of antagonizing the binding to RAGE could inhibit the harmful effects of AGEs. This antagonism could function through different means, such as inhibiting RAGE expression, interfering with intracellular signaling mediated by RAGE, or increasing the plasma levels of the circulating sRAGE, given its ability to serve as a decoy receptor to trap AGEs [182,183]. Numerous existing agents have proven to reach these objectives; among the most remarkable are statins [184,185] and thiazolidinediones

[186]. Beyond their potential as a lipid-lowering agent [187] and an oral hypoglycemic agent, respectively [188], both have demonstrated an in vivo reduction of RAGE expression [184,185,186] in conjunction with increased serum levels of sRAGE. It has been suggested that said effects depend upon the activation of the peroxisome proliferator-activated receptor γ (PPAR-γ), which could inhibit the phosphorylation of ERK1/2 and, thus, suppress the activation of NF-KB, decreasing the expression of both proinflammatory cytokines and RAGE [189,190]. Moreover, azeliragon (PF-04494700 or TTP488), an oral antagonist of RAGE, has obtained favorable results in animal models of Alzheimer's disease and was proven safe and effective at low doses in diverse clinical trials [191,192] (NCT02080364), being established as a promising therapeutic agent in the management of chronic complications of DM such as diabetic retinopathy [193].

Other molecules being widely researched are glucagon-like peptide-1 (GLP-1) and its analog exendin-4. Various experimental studies have shown their ability to decrease RAGE expression by suppressing NF-KB and reducing ROS generation by decreasing NADPH oxidase activity [194,195]. Consequently, these results have been associated with reducing the damage related to the activation of the AGE–RAGE axis in diseases like diabetic retinopathy [196], atherosclerosis

[197], and diabetic cardiomyopathy [198].

Go to:

7. Future Perspectives

The clinical potential of these interventions has not been completely established yet. For instance, aminoguanidine, despite being the first drug capable of examining the concept that inhibiting the formation of AGEs could lead to a clinically significant attenuation of a severe complication of diabetes [199], had to be suspended due to drug safety issues secondary to multiple adverse effects, such as its prooxidative potential [200], inhibition of NO synthase [201], abnormalities in liver function, development of antineutrophil cytoplasm antibodies, and even some cases of glomerulonephritis [145].

However, some agents, including alagebrium, benfotiamine, pyridoxamine, and thiazolidinediones, have achieved promising results in recent clinical trials [130,131,132,133,134,135,136,202,203,204]. Nonetheless, there are no available therapies specifically directed to prevent or eradicate AGEs; most of the preliminary clinical trials have focused on assessing the single effect of any particular AGE inhibitor, excluding the rest of the signaling pathways that could be intervened. Respectively, it would be excellent to research the combined effect of two or more inhibitors that act on different steps of the AGE–RAGE axis. Additionally, designing a drug with a broad spectrum of action to obtain better results in controlling the adverse effects of AGEs in the organism can be a further alternative.

In this sense, sRAGE has emerged as a promising molecule to competitively inhibit RAGE activation, modulating the systemic inflammation produced by the AGE–RAGE axis in multiple experimental studies. [205]. By acting as a decoy for RAGE ligands, sRAGE is able to attenuate inflammatory signaling, oxidative stress, and metabolic dysregulation. However, these findings came from experimental models [206].

Go to:

8. Conclusions

The action of AGEs in the development of chronic complications of DM has been reported. The increase in plasma concentrations of AGEs, either due to an increase in their consumption or due to their intrinsic formation, as well as the subsequent activation of RAGE, is known as the AGE–RAGE axis, which functions as a powerful inducer of proinflammatory pathways by promoting the synthesis of cytokines such as TNF-α, IL, VCAM-1, and even the increase of ROS, which has harmful effects on the micro- and macrovasculature of the target organs affected in DM. As a result, the interest in AGEs as a therapeutic target has increased, with the aim of creating drugs that can interfere with the activity of these molecules, decrease their concentration, or antagonize the AGE–RAGE axis, opening up the possibility of finding a new way to reduce the damage in target organs and improve the quality of life of patients. Additionally, the measurement of AGEs has acquired relevance, since they can be considered better markers than HbA1c. Studies using the SAF assessment have shown that increased levels are related to the risk factors of long-term complications; thus, these noninvasive tools could be used to establish the risk of developing DM complications, allowing for prompt intervention.

The role of glycation in the pathogenesis of aging and its prevention through herbal products and physical exercise

Chan-Sik Kim,1 Sok Park,2 and Junghyun Kim3,*
Author information Article notes Copyright and License information PMC Disclaimer

Go to:

Abstract

[Purpose]

Advanced glycation end products (AGEs) are non-enzymatic modifications of proteins or lipids after exposure to sugars. In this review, the glycation process and AGEs are introduced, and the harmful effects of AGEs in the aging process are discussed.

[Methods]

Results from human and animal studies examining the mechanisms and effects of AGEs are considered. In addition, publications addressing means to attenuate glycation stress through AGE inhibitors or physical exercise are reviewed.

[Results]

AGEs form in hyperglycemic conditions and/ or the natural process of aging. Numerous publications have demonstrated acceleration of the aging process by AGEs. Exogenous AGEs in dietary foods also trigger organ dysfunction and tissue aging. Various herbal supplements or regular physical exercise have beneficial effects on glycemic control and oxidative stress with a consequent reduction of AGE accumulation during aging.

[Conclusion]

The inhibition of AGE formation and accumulation in tissues can lead to an increase in lifespan.

Keywords: Advanced glycation end products, Aging, Glycation, Herbal products, Physical exercise

Go to:

INTRODUCTION

Aging is defined as a progressive loss of the efficacy of biochemical and physiological processes that occur until death[1]. A number of theories have been introduced to explain the aging process. One theory is that the abnormal accumulation of biological waste products in the organism is responsible for organ or tissues senescence[2, 3].

Glycation is a spontaneous non-enzymatic reaction of free reducing sugars with free amino groups of proteins, DNA, and lipids that forms Amadori products. The Amadori products undergo a variety of irreversible dehydration and rearrangement reactions that lead to the formation of advanced glycation end products (AGEs). This process was first introduced by Louis-Camille Maillard in 1912[4]. The glycation process leads to a loss of protein function and impaired elasticity of tissues such as blood vessels, skin, and tendons[5-7]. The glycation reaction is highly accelerated in the presence of hyperglycemia and tissue oxidative stress[8]. This implicates it in the pathogenesis of diabetic complications and aging[9]. Because there are no enzymes to remove glycated products from the human body, the glycation process matches well with the theory that the accumulation of metabolic waste promotes aging.

Oxidative stress has a very important role in the mechanism by which AGEs form and accumulate, and has been implicated as a key factor in the progression of various diseases, including chronic diseases such as diabetes, Alzheimer's disease, and aging[10-12]. Oxidative stress, more specifically oxidative damage to proteins, is increasingly thought to play a central mechanistic role in this context, as it is associated with modifications in the activities of biological compounds and cellular processes that may be linked to a pathological environment. Oxidative stress is fueled by the generation of excessive reactive oxygen species

(ROS) from glucose autoxidation, and also the nonenzymatic, covalent attachment of glucose molecules to circulating proteins that result in the formation of AGEs[13].

Naturally occurring phytochemicals and products are relatively safe for human consumption as compared to synthetic compounds, and are relatively inexpensive and available in orally ingestible forms. The search for an inhibitor of AGE formation has identified several natural products that prevent the glycation process. A number of medical herbs, dietary plants, and phytocompounds inhibit protein glycation both in vitro and in vivo[14]. These natural products with high antioxidant capacity may be promising agents for the prevention of glycation and AGE formation. Their anti-AGE activity may be one mechanism of their beneficial actions on human health[15].

Numerous previous reports indicate that the gradual decrease in systemic antioxidant capacity is the casuse of biological aging[16]. Other evidence supports the wide consensus that physical exercise improves systemic antioxidant activity[17]. Physical exercise can decrease oxidative stress in rodent animal models[18, 19]. Moderate physical exercise induces the expression of antioxidant enzymes, leading to the reduction of oxidative stress[20]. Additionally, regular physical exercise reduces AGE levels in renal tissues of obese Zucker rats[21] and has a beneficial effect on glycemic control in patients with diabetes[22]. Therefore, physical exercise may be a powerful weapon against AGE formation and AGE-related aging processes.

In this review, we discuss the implication of AGEs on the aging process. We also consider the potential inhibitory activity of herbal products and physical exercise in age-related organ dysfunction induced by glycation and/or AGEs, and the underling mechanisms.

Go to:

DEFINITION of GLYCATION and AGEs

AGEs were initially identified in the cooking process as the result of a nonenzymatic reaction between sugars and proteins within foods; this reaction is called the Maillard reaction[4]. The glycation process is initiated by a chemical reaction between the reactive carbonyl group of a sugar or an aldehyde with a nucleophilic free amino group of a protein, leading to the rapid formation of an unstable Schiff base. This adduct then undergoes rearrangement to form a reversible and more stable Amadori product. These intermediate products undergo further irreversible oxidation, dehydration, polymerization, and cross-linking reactions resulting in the formation of AGEs over the course of several days to weeks (Figure 1). Some important AGE compounds are shown in Figure 2.

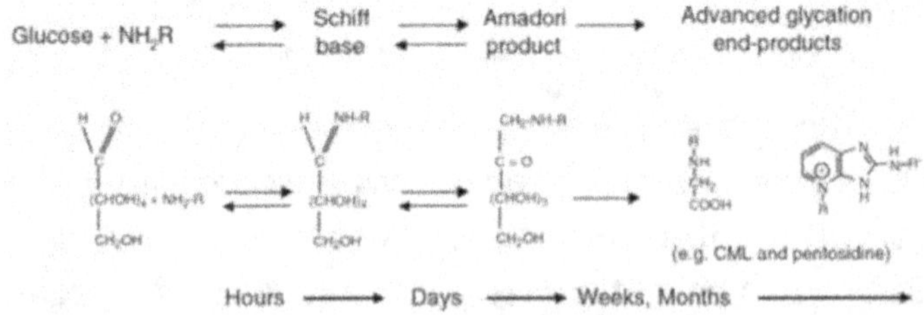

Figure 1.
Glycation process leading to the formation of advanced glycation end-products (AGEs). Illustration from Bohlender et al., 2005.

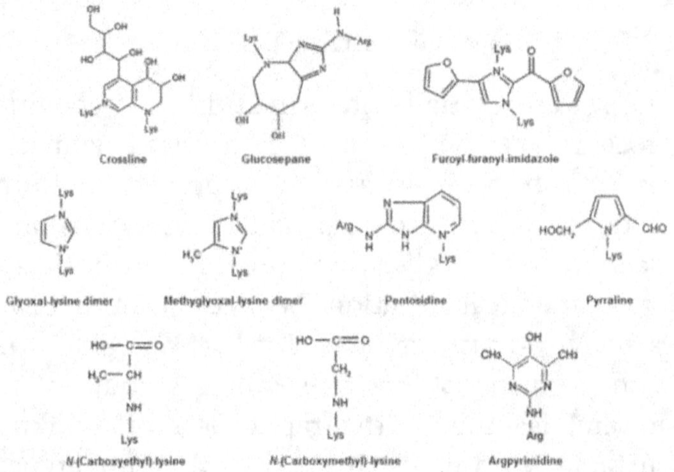

Figure 2.
Examples of biologically relevant advanced glycation end-products (AGEs). Illustration from Sadowska-Bartoz and Bartosz, 2016.

Go to:

ROLE of AGEs DURING AGING

The accumulation of glycated macromolecules, including proteins, is a hallmark of aging both in humans and experimental animals. The accumulation of AGEs was shown in Drosophila melanogaster and Caenorhabditis elegans. The content of AGEs in young (10 days old) D. melanogaster flies is 44% lower than in senescent (75 days old) flies[23]. C. elegans grown under high glucose conditions (40 mM) have a shortened lifespan and increased AGE content[24]. **Table 1** shows the available evidence for the accumulation of AGEs during aging and in different pathologies.

Table 1.

AGE accumulation in tissues during aging.

Tissue	AGEs	Commentary	Reference
Heart	CML	Increase with age	68
Lamina cribrosa	Pentosidine	Increase with age	69
Lung collagen	Pentosidine	Increase with age	70
Patellar tendon	Pentosidine	Increase with age	62
Skin	Argpyrimidine	Increase	71

	Pentosidine	with age	
Vitreous body	Pentosidine	Accumulation with age	72
Oocytes	Pentosidine	Increase with age	73
Intervertebral disk	Pentosidine	Increase with age	74
Cartilage	Pentosidine CEL, CML	Increase with age	75

Open in a separate window

CEL, *N*-(carboxyethyl)-lysine; CML, *N*-(carboxymethyl)-lysine.

Glycation is one of the endogenous aging mechanisms that occurs spontaneously with time, but also in a pathological manner during diabetes, renal failure, and inflammation[25]. AGEs are highly accumulated in tissues and organs in numerous age-related degenerative diseases. These toxic adducts (glycotoxins) are implicated in cell dysfunction, especially in diabetic patients and older organisms. AGE formation and accumulation in diabetic patients results in vascular alterations leading to diabetic vasculopathy.

There are three major mechanisms by which AGEs induce injury to the extracellular matrix (ECM) and cells, thereby contributing to aging and age-related diseases: (1) accumulation of AGEs within the ECM (such as collagen and elastic fibers) and cross-linking between AGEs and ECM causing a decrease in connective tissue elasticity, (2) glycated modifications of intracellular proteins causing a loss of the original cellular function, and (3) interaction of AGEs with their cellular receptor (RAGE), leading to the subsequent activation of inflammatory signaling pathways, ROS generation, and apoptosis[26].

Glycation of extracellular proteins induces the cross-linking of collagen and elastic fibers. As a consequence, elasticity of the ECM is altered, affecting especially vascular functions. There is a marked correlation between the serum concentration of N-(carboxymethyl)-lysine (CML) and vessel stiffness in elderly individuals[27]. Altering the balance between synthesis and degradation of ECM by glycated modifications may accelerate skin aging and increase skin stiffness[28]. Furthermore, cross-linking between AGEs and collagen impairs the mechanical properties of collagen. In particular, the cross-linking of AGEs with collagen of the vascular wall alters its structure and function, facilitating plaque formation and basement membrane hyperplasia[29].

Glycation also affects intracellular proteins. Intracellular AGE-modification of signaling molecules may impair cellular functions and gene expression[30]. For example, the activities of several antioxidant enzymes, including catalase, glutathione peroxidase, and glutathione reductase, are reduced by glycated modifications. Alterations of these enzyme activities increases cellular oxidative stress[31, 32]. In addition, glycated proteins are usually removed via ubiquitin-dependent 20S proteasome-mediated proteolysis. AGE-modifications can disturb this proteolytic degradation, contributing to a further increase in the cellular content of glycated proteins[33].

RAGE is the best-characterized cell surface molecule that recognizes AGEs. The interaction between an AGE and its receptor alters cell and organ functions mainly through inflammatory molecules, leading to aging. RAGE regulates a number of cell processes of crucial importance such as inflammation, apoptosis, ROS signaling, proliferation, autophagy, and aging[34, 35].

Go to:

DIETARY AGEs

Endogenous glycation reactions occur spontaneously with a small proportion of intestinally absorbed sugars[36]. However, food is an important source of exogenous AGEs. The role of dietary AGEs and their interaction with RAGE during aging has been demonstrated recently[37]. The Maillard reaction is often used to improve the color, flavor, aroma, and texture of foods. However, significant generation of AGEs occurs when sugars are cooked with proteins[38].

In a mouse model, feeding an AGE-rich diet for 16 weeks promoted a 53% increase in the serum levels of AGEs[39]. Uribarri et al. reported that, in renal failure patients, there was a 29% increase in CML levels in the blood of those subjected to an AGE-rich diet, while a 34% reduction of CML was detected in the group fed a low AGE diet[40]. In a mouse model, a 9-month dietary exposure to CML accelerated endothelial dysfunction and arterial aging. These results suggest that a diet restricting AGEs could be an effective way to reduce the AGE burden in the human body.

Go to:

AGE INHIBITORS

There is considerable interest in the therapeutic potential of agents that can inhibit the formation of AGEs or break AGE-mediated cross-links[41, 42]. Several synthetic or natural agents have been proposed as AGE inhibitors.

Aminoguanidine was first introduced as an AGE inhibitor[43]. AGE inhibitors, including aminoguanidine and pyridoxamine, prevent AGE accumulation by interacting with the highly reactive carbonyl species and acting as carbonyl traps[44, 45]. In previous reports, aminoguanidine prevented diabetic renal, retinal, and neural complications through the inhibition of AGE formation[46]. However, due to safety concerns resulting from its adverse effects, including pro-oxidant activities[47] and inhibition of NO synthase[48], aminoguanidine cannot be used clinically[49].

Recently, several researchers have suggested that a novel agent can destroy preformed AGE-derived protein cross-links. The first identified AGE breaker, N-phenacylthiazolium bromide, was introduced in 1996. Because N-phenacylthiazolium bromide is unstable in vitro, it was not clinically successful. Another compound, alagebrium[50], was developed as an AGE breaker. Alagebrium could reverse AGE accumulation in vivo[51]. However, clinical studies on these compounds were terminated and none of the known AGE breakers are in clinical use.

Herbal products are generally recognized as relatively safe for human consumption, compared with synthetic drugs. Thus, the search for anti-AGE agents using herbal products has been increasing[52]. Many herbal products have potent anti-glycation activities, and these activities are similar or even stronger than aminoguanidine. For example, several polyphenols can inhibit the glycation process in vitro. Flavonoids are the major class of polyphenols. Anti-glycation properties of various flavonoids, such as kaempferol, genistein, quercitrin, and quercetin, have been reported[53-56]. Recently, we demonstrated a potent AGE breaking property of epicatechin in vitro and in vivo. This compound destroyed preformed glycated serum albumin in vitro and decreased AGE accumulation in retinal tissues of rats injected with exogenous AGE[42]. In the AGE structure, side chains attached to the pyrrole ring carbons are susceptible to nucleophilic attack[57]. Because C6 and C8 on the A-ring of epicatechin are nucleophilic[58], epicatechin can attack and destroy the AGE cross-links.

Go to:
EFFECT of PHYSICAL EXERCISE on AGEs

Many previous reports have shown the ability of physical activity to improve glycemic control, with a consequent reduction of AGE accumulation in diabetic patients and during aging[36, 59]. In a rat model, 12 weeks of moderate physical exercise reduced the contents of CML and RAGE in aortic vessels[60]. Another study showed that rats subjected to treadmill exercise from late middle age to 35 months old had reduced AGE levels in cardiac tissues compared to age-matched control animals[61]. In human subjects, life-long trained athletes had 21% lower contents of AGE cross-links in the patellar tendon compared to age-matched untrained subjects[62]. Recently, we also showed the positive effect of regular exercise on the renal accumulation of AGEs. Specifically, regular exercise significantly prevented renal AGE deposition in D-galactose-induced aging rats. We also showed that treadmill exercise reduced CML accumulation and had retinoprotective effects in naturally-aged mice[63].

Regular physical activity has beneficial contributions to physical capacity, hypertension, oxidative stress, and lipid metabolism[64, 65]. Especially, physical exercise effectively inhibits ROS generation and improves the activities of antioxidant enzymes[66]. The higher energy demands induced by physical exercise might reduce the pool of reactive intermediates available for glycation[21]. Because the protein glycation reaction is driven and accelerated by ROS, the inhibition of AGE formation by regular exercise may be the main mechanism of exercise-associated antioxidant activity. Additionally, AGE formation can be retarded or attenuated through efficient glycemic control[67]. Therefore, it can be assumed that regular physical exercise also can improve glycemic control, which attenuates the formation and accumulation of AGEs in tissues.

Go to:

CONCLUSION

In this review, we provide insights into the anti-glycation activities of herbal products and physical exercise. There is extensive scientific evidence documenting the accumulation of AGEs with aging and age-related diseases. Thus, we suggest that inhibiting the glycation process and removing existing glycation products may prolong the lifespan. In this sense, dietary herbal supplements or physiological exercise may be distinctly advantageous in reducing the burden of AGEs in our body.

TECHNOLOGY EQUIPMENT RECAP

<u>Melanocytes</u> - Photovoltaic Cells

<u>Neurons/Nerves</u> - Electromagnetic Cells

<u>Fascia</u> - Plasma Medium (misonomered Ether)

<u>Brain</u> - CPU, Inductor

<u>Brainstem</u> - Two-way Adapter for CPU into the Motherboard

<u>Pineal Gland</u> - Receiver, Crystal Tuner & Actuator Arm/Head responsible for Phosphorescence, Thermoluminescence, Piezoelectricity, Birefringence & Harmonic Generation (very much like the otoconia in the ears)

<u>Operating System</u> - Deductive Logic or PQ

<u>Heart</u> - Hydraulic Ram, Turbine (from the Greek τύρβη, tyrbē, or Latin turbo, meaning vortex) and

Hard Drive.

<u>Melanosomes</u> - Alternators

<u>Mitochondria</u> - Motors

<u>Myelin Sheath</u> - Insulation

<u>Cytoskeleton</u> - Filaments

<u>Phospholipids</u> - Capacitors, Dielectric Material (lipids in general)

<u>Spine</u> - Piezoelectric, Motherboard, Radio Wave Antenna

<u>RBC</u> - Floppy Discs

<u>Lymph Nodes</u> - Filters, Nodes

<u>Protein</u> - Transformer

<u>Transformers 'Roll Out'</u> - Conformational Change (Macromolecule Shape Shifting)

<u>Antioxidants</u> - Semi-conductors (especially the selenium based...)

<u>Body Cells</u> - Plasma based Crystal disc, fitted with integrated circuits as well as gates and channels (see Human Cell Membrane and/or Computer Chip)

<u>Nerves & Vessels</u> - 'Copper' wires (CoAxial Cables) and Fiber Optics

<u>Pigment, Nerve & Blood Clusters</u> - Input Devices like a Mouse, Keyboard, etc...

<u>DNA</u> - Piezoelectric, Antenna, Data Storing Inductors.

<u>Collagen Based Tissue</u> - Piezoelectric Inductors

<u>Stomach</u> - Chemical Mixer

Lumen - the SI unit of luminous flux = to the amount of light emitted per second..... or hollow structures in vessels and cells... hmmm????

Eyes - Camera Lens/Charge Coupled Device (CCD), Digital to Analogue Converter, Complex Photovoltaic Cells/Photodetector...

Amino Acids - Fuses that can be almost anything!

Nucleic Acid - Actual Intelligence (self powering too).

N-Type Semiconductors - Selenium or Silica doped with Phosphorus (Alkaline-ish)

P-Type Semiconductors - Selenium or Silica doped with Boron (Acid-ish)

PN Junction - <u>Crystal Lattice Structure</u> Material allowing the flowing of electrons in one direction.

Bone and Fascia seem to be a massive N-Type, P-Type, PN Junction Super computer on it's own... especially if we add in the Piezoelectricity & Vitamin D!

Melanin - CPU Core, Solar Repeater

Human Cell Membrane and/or Computer Chip - A flat semiconducting (crystal) disc or wafer, with integrated circuits (resistors/conductors) and/or gates & channels. We now have to add the filaments into this Crystal Disc we call a Body Cell or Somatic Cell.

Transistors - a semiconductor device with three connections, capable of amplification in addition to rectification.

The location that a virus goes viral in, is called a

Hotspot? WTH!

Virus - an infective agent that typically consists of a nucleic acid molecule in a protein coat, is too small to be seen by light microscopy, and is able to multiply only within the living cells of a host.

Wait you see that, it is happening again! Host...

See look there is another definition of **Virus** - a piece of code that is capable of copying itself and typically has a detrimental effect, such as corrupting the system or destroying data.

Wait a damn minute! DNA is a piece of **code**... A viral strand of DNA or RNA that can jump host is fully capable in that context of copying itself, one would even argue, that is it's only 'motion'. The detrimental effects of corrupting the system (physical illness) or destroying data (mental illness), can clearly be seen anthropomorphically.

Host - an animal or plant on or in which a parasite or commensal organism lives. VS

Host - store (a website or other data) on a server or other computer so that it can be accessed over the internet.

Transmission is the act of transferring something from one spot to another, like a radio or TV broadcast, or a disease going from one person to another.

I am highlighting the unknown and proposing we may have some answers! <u>Infection - an infectious disease.</u>

plural noun: infections "a chest infection"

Vs

Infection - the presence of a virus in, or its introduction into, a computer system. What is a computer system?

<u>Computer System</u> - a computer system is a programmable electronic device that can accept input; store data; and retrieve, process and output information.

<u>Pandemic language = Virology/Biology language.</u> The question is, why? The next question is what does that have to do with Dr. Sebi or Robert Becker? The obvious....

<u>Computer System</u> - a computer system is a programmable electronic device that can accept input; store data; and retrieve, process and output information.

<u>Computer System</u> - a single information processor but usually a group of processors that have specified and general computations; grouped by hardware ie... liver cells, lung cells, brain cells etc.. What you think?

<u>Exercise</u> - activity requiring physical effort, carried out to sustain or improve health and fitness.
"exercise improves your heart and lung power"

<u>Exercise</u> - computer training or computer based training.

<u>Resonance</u> - the quality in a sound of being deep, full, and reverberating. "the resonance of his voice"

- The ability to evoke or suggest images, memories, and emotions."the concepts lose their emotional resonance"

- The reinforcement or prolongation of sound

by reflection from a surface or by the synchronous vibration of a neighboring object.

- The condition in which an electric circuit or device produces the largest possible response to an applied oscillating signal, especially when its inductive and its capacitative reactances are balanced.

- The condition in which an object or system is subjected to an oscillating force having a frequency close to its own natural frequency.

- The occurrence of a simple ratio between the periods of revolution of two bodies about a single primary.

- The state attributed to certain molecules of having a structure that cannot adequately be represented by a single structural formula but is a composite of two or more structures of higher energy.

- • A short-lived subatomic particle that is an excited state of a more stable particle.

Induction - the action or process of inducting someone to a position or organization."the league's induction into the Baseball Hall of Fame"

Induction - a formal introduction to a new job or position.plural noun: inductions
"an induction course"
enlistment into military service.

Induction - The process or action of bringing about or giving rise to something."isolation, starvation, and other forms of stress induction" the process of bringing on childbirth or abortion by artificial means, typically by the use of drugs.

Induction - The inference of a general law from particular instances.

Induction -"the admission that laws of nature cannot be established by induction" the production of facts to prove a general statement.

Induction - a means of proving a theorem by showing that if it is true of any particular case it is true of the next case in a series, and then showing that it is indeed true in one particular case.

Induction - noun: mathematical induction; plural noun: mathematicals inductionthe production of an electric or magnetic state by the proximity (without contact) of an electrified or magnetized body.

Induction - The production of an electric current in a conductor by varying the magnetic field applied to the conductor.

Induction - The stage of the working cycle of an internal combustion engine in which the fuel mixture is drawn into the cylinders.

Is there anyone reading this that would disagree with

our body fitting these definitions, the definitions of a computer?

Man this thought experiment just got a lot more interesting didn't it? MIT and the US Military are different types of receipts huh? Is it possible frequency resonance, spreads disease? Human modems? Can Shedding be a broadcast signal?

Wi-Fi is a wireless networking technology that uses radio waves to provide wireless high-speed Internet access. A common misconception is that the term **Wi-Fi** is short for "wireless fidelity," however Wi-Fi is a trademarked phrase that refers to IEEE 802.11x standards.

Viral shedding is a term for when viruses are replicating or reproducing, the virus is being led out of the host cell where it's replicating or

reproducing ... Viral shedding is the expulsion and release of virus progeny following successful reproduction during a host cell infection. Once replication has been completed and the host cell is exhausted of all resources in making viral progeny, the viruses may begin to leave the cell by several methods.

Vaccine - a substance used to stimulate immunity to a particular infectious disease or pathogen, typically prepared from

an inactivated or weakened form of the causative agent or from

its constituents or products.

Vaccine - a program designed to detect computer viruses and inactivate them.

"the rate of use of vaccines for computer viruses is not as high as in the US, Japan, and other countries"

<u>Application</u> - a medicinal substance put on the skin.

<u>Application</u> - a program or piece of software designed and written to fulfill a particular purpose of the user.

In our thought experiment, if a virus is simply the media for harmful information...

<u>Media</u> - an intermediate layer in the wall of a blood vessel or lymphatic vessel.

<u>Media</u> - the main means of mass communication (broadcasting, publishing, and the internet) regarded collectively.

<u>DOPE</u> - an illicit drug (such as heroin or cocaine) used for its intoxicating or euphoric effects
especially : MARIJUANA (dopamine altering)

<u>Dope</u> - a preparation (such as an anabolic steroid, diuretic, or tranquilizer) given to a racehorse to help or hinder its performance

<u>To Dope</u> - In semiconductor production, to dope is the intentional introduction of impurities into an intrinsic semiconductor for the purpose of modulating its electrical, optical and structural properties. The doped material is referred to as an extrinsic semiconductor.

<u>Short Circuit</u> - Cardiac Arrest?

<u>Short Circuit</u> - Multiple Sclerosis (due to loss of insulation)

<u>Overheating</u> - Fever?

<u>Overcurrent</u> - Inflammation

With Infection and Virus included we are onto something.

<u>Current</u> - belonging to the present time; happening or being used or done now.

<u>Current</u> - *a body of water* or air *moving in a definite direction*, especially *through a surrounding body of water* or air in which there is less movement.

<u>Current</u> - a flow of electricity that results from the ordered directional movement of electrically charged particles.

<u>Current</u> - a quantity representing the rate of flow of electric charge, usually measured in amperes.

<u>Current</u> - the general tendency or course of events or opinion.

<u>Leakage Current</u> - the unintended loss of energy, gain of resistance or results of faulty/worn out insulation.

<u>Plasma</u> - Electric Currents or Electric Current Carrier

<u>Electric Current</u> - Magnetic Field (AtomSphere) Carrier

<u>Alternating Magnetic & Electric Waves</u> - Light

<u>NeuroTransmitters</u> - Record of ElectroMagnetic Waves produced by Neurons (ElectroChemical Message)

<u>Hormones</u> - Large simple versions of NeuroTransmitters (ElectroChemical Message)

<u>Malware</u> - External Negative Mental Programming

<u>Food</u> - Informative Electronic Batteries

<u>Conductor</u> - a person who directs the performance of an orchestra or choir.

<u>Conductor</u> - a material or device

that conducts or transmits heat, electricity, or sound, especially when regarded in terms of its capacity to do this.

Lymphatic System - Watermill

Circulatory System - Generator

Integumentary System - Photovoltaic Diaphragm

Immune System - Antivirus, Malware Scanner, Frequency Filter & Rectifier

Nervous System - Power Transmission and Cellular Communications Lines

Fascia System - HydroElectric Grid

Respiratory System - Windmill

Windmill - a structure that converts wind power or "air" power into rotational energy or vortex energy, to mill grain. In our case grain is Magnetism!

MAGNETS ARE DEFINED BY GRAINS
MAGNETIC GRAINS ARE DEFINED BY APPLIED
STRESS AND CRYSTAL GEOMETRY
SPM SUPERMAGNETIC
SD SINGLE DOMAIN
PSD PSEUDO DOMAIN
MD MULTIDOMAIN

Reproductive System - Quine (self-replicating programs)

Skeletal System - Piezoelectric Crystal Shaped to produced highly specific frequency under stress, Dynamic Oscillators.

Urinary System - Industrial Wastewater, Return Flow,

Surface Runoff, Urban Runoff Agricultural & Animal Husbandry Wastewater

Digestive System - Massive Inductor

Mouth - Industrial Grinder

Endocrine System - Programmer for Human Cell Membrane and/or Crystal Gel Computer Chips

Human Being - Resonator

Vessels - Pipes

Aromatic Ring - Cyclotron (Particle Accelerator)

Glycation - Corrosion

GLOSSARY

anode - electrode where the oxidation half-reaction takes place

battery - galvanic cell in which the electrical work is used as a source of electrical power

cathode - electrode where the reduction half-reaction takes place

cathodic protection - method of protecting a metal by sacrificing another metal as an anode in a galvanic cell

circuit - path through which electrons flow

corrosion - process by which metals oxidize and return from a reduced form to their natural oxidation state

dry cell - galvanic cell in which the electrolytes exist as pastes

electric current - flow of electric charge

electric potential - amount of work required to move one charged particle from one point to another

electrical work - voltage between two points when a charged particle is moved between them

electrochemistry - branch of science that studies chemical reactions that cause electrons to move, resulting in the transfer of electrical charge

electrode - electrical conductor through which current enters or leaves an electrochemical cell

electrolysis - process of using electric current to do work on a chemical cell against its electric potential

electrolyte - ionic solution that can be decomposed by electricity

electrolytic cell - electrochemical cell that requires electrical energy to drive a nonspontaneous redox reaction

Faraday constant - charge of one mole of electrons (96,485 C/mol)

fuel cell - device that generates electrical power through the ionization of hydrogen or another molecule

galvanic cell - electrochemical cell formed when metal strips connected by a wire are immersed in different solutions of a redox reaction and the solutions are connected by a salt bridge

galvanic cell notation - shorthand method of describing the setup of a galvanic cell

galvanization - process that coats a metal with zinc as a sacrificial anode

inert electrode - electrode that does not take part in a chemical reaction but serves only to transfer electrons

Nernst equation - equation used to find the cell potential under conditions that are not standard.

oxidation half-reaction - half-reaction showing oxidation (electron loss) of a species

reduction half-reaction - half-reaction showing reduction (electron gain) of a species

sacrificial anode - anode made of a metal coupled to a more valuable metal, which it protects as part of a galvanic cell that undergoes galvanic corrosion

salt bridge - inert connection between the two half-cells, composed of either a glass tube filled with an inert salt solution or a strip of filter paper soaked in an inert salt solution, that transfers ions between the half-cells

standard cell potential - potential difference between

the cathode and the anode under standard conditions

standard hydrogen electrode (SHE) - platinum electrode in 1 M H+(aq) solution with bubbled hydrogen gas at 1 atm of pressure

standard reduction potential (E°) - tendency of the species to be reduced under standard conditions

RUN THAT BY ME AGAIN

Glucose + Oxygen -----> Carbon dioxide + Water + Energy

or

$$C_6H_{12}O_6 + 6O_2 \longrightarrow 6CO_2 + 6H_2O + 2900 \text{ kj}$$

When doing the exercises outlined in the gold book, your body increases the unloading of O_2 from hemoglobin to myoglobin in the working muscle, increase AMP synthesis, reroutes the blood flow to the skeletal muscles form non-essential organs (stimulate EPO in the kidneys), increase breath rate and heart rate.

This speeds up all chemical reactions which lead to a massive boost in BMR, that boost in BMR can be used to excite the mTOR system or the Longevity System. This is why the Dopamine, Serotonin, Beta Endorphins and Endocannabinoids are all unregulated to get you high, make the pain of exercise feel addictive!

Glycation goes with C-Reactive Proteins eventually leading to Troponin (the new slow death).

It's funny how we started with Iodine and now we are gonna discuss Irish moss, just kidding but that may help your remember Irisin.

Irisin - named after Iris, the Greek messenger goddess a 112-amino-acid peptide, turns white adipocytes into brown adipocytes, adds bone density and repairs nerve function. This is the most powerful health transforming Myokine to date. Irisin regulates some risk factors of AD (Alzheimer's disease), which includes altered neurogenesis, oxidative stress, insulin resistance, and imbalance of neurotrophic factors.

Myokine - Cytokines produced by muscles to communicate with the other cells and of course Melanocytes. Irisin is also produced by smooth muscles ie the Pancreas, Liver...

AMPK stimulates the release of Irisin...

Lets run the scrimmage now..

You get off your couch or stop masterbating, then you start the program in the Gold Book, Divine Mathematics Book and the AlgaRhythm Book.
Your Body Heat goes up, meaning the internal production of Light.

The CPU sends a signal through the Adapter to the Motherboard, Dilate the Dermal Blood Vessel and Activate the Sweat Glands.

You are now officially Radiating Light aka Body Heat.

The Sugars and Fats in the blood are all getting burned up...

You Relax..

Make a big smoothie with Agave, Dates, Mangos, Bananas, Sweet Grapes, Protein Powder and have a nice big meal…

You just blew it!

All that damn sugar Bwahahahahaha

You just loaded up on Glucose and Fructose….

Never use Agave! Dr. Sebi was half crazy telling people to use Agave syrup! Agave syrup is 90% Fructose!!!! Fructose uncoupled from Fiber, Pigments or Proteins, No!
That is how you successfully block AMPK, Melanin Concentrating Hormone and Autophagy! Let Dr. Sebi rest in Greatness, you can do that by realizing his food list was cool but it was created in the 70s and 80s. The painful thing is we still have't learned much in the last 50 years as a people. I hope these books change that, please join the fight against the idiocracy!

www.ingramcontent.com/pod-product-compliance
Lightning Source LLC
Chambersburg PA
CBHW061638250726

48659CB00004B/1283